Herbal Home Remedies

Published by :
Lotus Press Publishers & Distributors

Herbal Home Remedies

Dr. Rajeev Sharma
M.D., D.Lit.

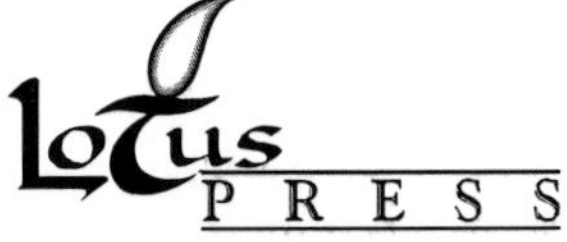

4735/22, Prakash Deep Building
Ansari Road, Darya Ganj,
New Delhi - 110002

Lotus Press : Publishers & Distributors
Unit No. 220, 2nd Floor, 4735/22, Prakash Deep Building,
Ansari Road, Darya Ganj, New Delhi- 110002
Ph.: 23280047, 98118-38000
• E-mail : lotuspress1984@gmail.com
www.lotuspress.co.in

Herbal Home Remedies

ISBN: 81-8382-054-9

Attention Readers:

Every effort is made to ensures accuracy of material, but the publisher, printer and author will not be held responsible for any inadvertent error(s). In case of any dispute, all legal matters to be settled under Delhi Jurisdiction only.

Printed & Published by : **Lotus Press Publishers & Distributors,** New Delhi-02

A brief about

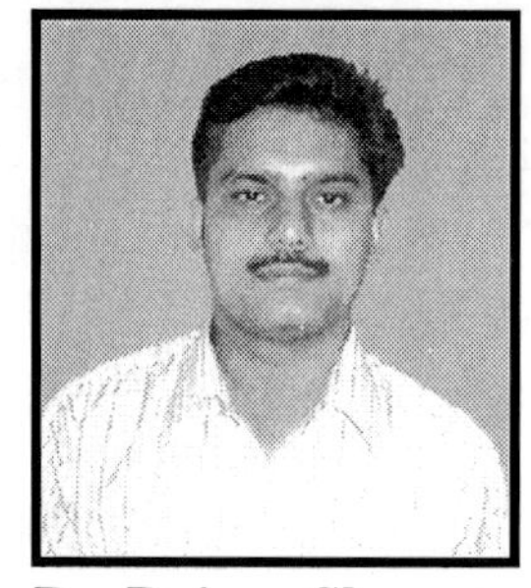

Dr. Rajeev Sharma

Dr. Rajeev Sharma is an eminent consultant of Homoeopathy, Yoga, Naturopathy and Alternative Medicine in India. He has written more than two hundred books in Hindi and English and around one thousand five hundred articles which have been published in various newspapers and magazines. He is also an Editional Board Member of the prestigious *Asian Homoeopathic Journal* besides many other newspapers and magazines.

Dr. Rajeev Sharma has written books on ayurveda, homoeopathy, yoga, naturopahty, accupressure, magnetotherapy, water-therapy, massage and aromatherapy etc.

Dr. Rajeev Sharma has written books on all major ailments like diabetes, hypertension, obesity, stomach and respiriatory disorders, E.N.T. disorders, female & male disorders, UTI disorders sexual disorders, paediatric problems, headache, stress and other mental problems.

The books written by Dr. Rajeev Sharma are published by renowned publishers of India.

Dr. Rajeev Sharma is Medical Advisor to Ralson Remedies (a homoeopathic medicines manufacturer), and Dixit Pharmacy (Ayurvedic Manufacturer), Medical Examiner at the Life Insurance Corporation of India. He has received several prizes for his outstanding achievements. He has been awarded the *Best Author* prize in Hindi by the Home Ministry and Ministry of Health and Family Welfare, Government of India and *Sarjana Puraskar* by U.P. Hindi Sansthan, Lucknow. He has delivered talks on All India Radio and lectures on Alternative Medicine in various government and non-government organisations. He has written at advertisement scripts for the products of several companies.

He is working as Educational Consultant and Marriage and Behaviour Counsellor too. He is a person of creative mind.

He has established an institute through which one can get certificates by correspondence in accupressure, massage, yoga water therapy, diet therapy, naturopathy, color therapy and reiki besides other paramedical courses.

He is providing literature on Personality Development and LIfe Style Management.

Dr. Rajeev Sharma is also a social activist. He has worked a lot against Addition and prevention of AIDS. Now a days, he is working to check the population growth of India with an NGO called 'Nav Chetna Manch'. He has worked for pollution control and human rights too and has received the World Human Rights Promotion Award. His name has been published in ***LIMCA BOOK OF RECORDS 2005***. He has developed two websites too:- *www.newkamasutra.com* and *www.indiaalive.net*

Preface

Herbs are those remedies which are natural and non-toxic. Most of the herbs have medicinal and curative properties. In past our rishi-munis were habitual of eating raw fruits and vegetables and their helath remained undisturbed even for hundred years. Fruits and vegetables are a part of herbal kingdom.

In this books I have included treatment by carrot, radish, ginger, onion, garlic, lemon, emblic myrobalan, turmeric, basil, margosa, bael, banana, dates, honey and water. There are separate chapters on fruits, vegetables and herbal tips too.

With the help of this book, you can treat your common ailments at home but always prefer a medical supervision.

Hundreds of diseases are covered by herbal home remedies. This is a family guide and from infant to old, everybody will be benefitted by this book.

Thanks

Dr. Rajeev Sharma
Srijan—AAROGYA JYOTI®
Palm—11/03, Shipra Suncity,
Indirapuram, Ghaziabad (UP)
Ph.: 0120-3020206
E-mail: sharmarajeev100@rediffmail.com

Contents

1

Your Health Guidelines

There is an interesting and important episode described in the text of *Ayurvedic Medicine*. While discussing with rishi Punarvasu, the author of *Charak Samhita*, some vaidyas (Ayurvedic doctors) raised the query *Ko'ruka*? (who does not fall ill?). Somebody said — one who eats *chyavanprash* every morning. "Who takes *lavan bhaskar* and *triphala* regularly" said some others; eating *chandravati* every day was described by another vaidya as the source of health. Finally the fundamental principle of natural maintenance of good health was expressed by Vagbhatt as—*"Hitbhuka, Mitbhuka, Ritbhuka". Hitbhuka:* means eat that which is nourishing for your health and do not eat merely for taste. *Mitbhuka:* means eat moderately (only that much which is essential for sustenance of the vitality and stamina of the body). *Ritbhuka:* means eat that which is earned and prepared by righteous means and also what is suitable in a particular season.

Broadly speaking, the above principles are not new to us. We all might have read or heard about these in one form or the other. But how many people (including ourselves) really pay due attention to these? In view of the life-style adopted by most of us today and considering the growing pollution in the gross and the subtle environment, we ought to be more careful about healthy food. This series is bringing us the pearls of knowledge from Ayurveda—the science of leading a long, happy and healthy life. In the last issue we had mentioned about the twelve categories of naturally nourishing food as described in the *Charak Samhita*. Here we look at these in detail to have some practical tips on what should we eat every day and how?

1. ***Shuka Grain (Cereals)***: Wheat, rice, barley, maize, millet, corn etc, are principal ingredients of Indian cooking. The cereals are natural sources of nourishment for human body. Carbohydrates are their major constituents. They also contain about 6 to 12 % proteins. The presence of minerals and vitamins is, however, nominal in the cereals; only vitamin B is found in greater quantity in their outer sheath. The shelf life of these cereals ranges between one to two years after harvesting. Sprouted cereals have more nutrition value and are richer in proteins and vitamins.
2. ***Shami Grains (Pulses and Legumes)***: This category of grains consists of grams and pulses, which are rich in proteins. Gram, green gram, kidney-beans,red and yellow gram and lentil, black-gram, soyabean seeds, drypeas, etc. fall in this category. These are main sources of proteins for vegetarians. The protein contents and mode of metabolism of these are healthier and more compatible with the metabolic functioning of the human body as compared to those in the non-vegetarian foods (meat, chicken, eggs etc). Use of fresh sprouts of whole pulses and legumes in balanced quantities in breakfast and main meals is an excellent means of maintaining natural health.
3. ***Kandamula (Tubers and Roots)***: Potato, sweet tuber (sweet potato), carrot, beetroot, turnip, radish, etc. are members of this class of naturally healthy foods. They are rich in carbohydrates and are important sources of balanced calories in our bodies and activation of metabolism. These, if eaten in appropriate quantities, are good means of strength and energy in the body system. These could even be used as substitutes for varieties of cereal dishes. The *rishi-munis* of the ancient times used to take only *kandamula* as their main food. The term *phalahara* for the food prescribed during fasts refers to these only.
4. ***Phal (Fruits)***: As we all know, vitamins, minerals, natural glucose and carbohydrates are present in substantial

proportions in fresh fruits. Amalki, apple, bilva (wood-apple), banana, black-plum (rose-apple), dates, figs, grapes, guava, mango, orange, pomegranate, papaya, sweet-lime, etc are easily available in India. According to Ayurveda, these fruits also have medicinal properties.Fruits like apricot, cherry, pineapple, strawberry; etc. could also be used. Ayurveda emphasizes that fruits should be eaten in their specific season, and should be naturally ripe. Over-ripe or rotten fruits are harmful. Raw fruits would be difficult to digest and will not have the desired natural qualities. Care should be taken to avoid eating fruits preserved in cold storage and those ripened through the use of chemicals like carbide. These have severe negative effects; frequent use of such unnaturally ripened fruits might cause dreaded diseases like cancer.

5. ***Shakas (Vegetables)***: Fresh vegetables are important ingredients of a healthy food. They provide us with essential vitamins, minerals and compounds. Use of different types of green beans, bitter gourd, brinjal, cabbage, cauliflower, cucumber, green-gourd, ladies-fingers,tomato, etc is very good for health. Different types of vegetables supplement each other in fulfilling the body's requirement of vitamins, minerals etc. Likewise the use of fruits, specific vegetables should also be consumed only in the specific season of their natural growth. Use of vegetables of one season in another season is prohibited in Ayurveda.
6. ***Harit (Greens Leafy Vegetables)***: Leaves of Coriander, fenugreek, green peas, mint, radish-leaf, spinach, etc. should be part of a healthy diet. Iron, calcium, and other minerals and vitamin C and E etc, present in these green leafy vegetables or salads, are essential for our body's proper nourishment.
7. ***Shuska Phal Va Tilahan (Dry Fruits and Oil Seeds)***: Almond, cashew nut, chestnut, coconut, groundnut, peanut, pistachio, etc are very rich in proteins. The oils inside these

provide natural lubricants and fats necessary for the body's mechanical and other functions. The edible, oily-seeds of seasamum, mustard, etc also serve this purpose.

8. ***Ikshu (Glucose Rich Substances)***: Molasses, sugarcane, sugar, treacle, and other glucose rich substances fall in this category. These are often used to sweeten the drinks and eatables. These contain hundred percent carbohydrates, which are the major source of producing energy in the body.
9. ***Ambu (Watery or Juicy Substances)***: This category includes all edible substances that are rich in water-content. Fruits like watermelon, which contain about 90% water, are prominent in this category. Major part of our body system is filled with water. We should fulfil the consistent requirement of its supply by drinking substantial amount of water. Fresh lemon squash, etc and juice of watery fruits, if taken in balanced quantities, also supply us with other nourishing substances along with water.
10. ***Goras (Milk products)***: Milk, curd, buttermilk, cheese, etc fall in this group. Pure milk (especially cow's) and buttermilk are described as 'divine' food or best source of nourishment for *sadhaks*. Many people observe *kalpa* (long-term fasting) only with the intake of milk or buttermilk. Milk (especially, cow's) is a whole food in itself. Curd is also nourishing food with several medicinal qualities, if taken fresh and in appropriate quantities in different seasons as per one's *prakrati* (level of *tridosha*). Fresh cheese and its products (if not fried) are wholesome sources of calories. Buttermilk *(takra)* is referred in Ayurveda as an important medicinal food. Condensed milk and milk powder might be easy to preserve and use, and may help in making delicious dishes, but these are harmful to health, particularly in the cozy life-style we have adopted and because of the chemical synthesis processes used in their preparation. Use of condensed milk and milk powder or dairy whiteners should therefore be avoided as far as possible. In view of the reports of adulteration of milk by mixing urea and other

chemicals, contaminated water, etc, these days, we should be careful in verifying and ascertaining that milk and its products are free from toxins.

11. ***Sneha (Oils and Fats)***: Butter, *ghee* (butter clarified by boiling and straining), edible oils and fatty substances, if taken in balanced amounts, are also part of a healthy diet. These are highly rich in calories. (On an average, about nine calories are gained from one gm of any of these substances). These help in fulfilling the requirements of lubrication of body parts (especially, joints) and energy production in the body-system. They also contain vitamins A, D, E and K. However, excess use of these substances is harmful to both physical and mental health. Extra care should therefore be taken to keep the level of proportion of this category to the essential minimum in our daily meals.

12. ***Krattana Va Yaugika (Cooked Food and Edible Compounds)***: Ayurveda considers 'cooked food' as a separate class of food. All the categories described above are independent of each other and, as we know, most of the constituents of these could be consumed raw or sprouted. Cooking changes the natural properties of food ingredients. However, eating this class of food is important because proper cooking (esp. of cereals and pulses) makes the food easily digestible and many of the new edible compounds produced under this process would also be of vital use in the metabolic system and other functions of the body. Cooked food could consist of members of more than one of the above classes and help giving new combined positive effects. The concept of cooking as referred in Ayurveda is quite different from what it is for most of us today.

Cooking today is mostly aimed to make the food more delicious; different experiments are tried out by the catering experts in this regard and ever new 'dishes' and new recipes are derived. Deep fried food, varieties of spices and arbitrary combination of foods of non-compatible natural qualities are harmful to our health according to Ayurveda. But we don't think of it as long as the food is palatable. The use of pre-cooked food-ingredients and the so-called "fast foods" should be avoided, as it has adverse effects on our body. Apart from lacking in nourishing value this type of 'modern' food is likely to impair the normal functioning of digestive system and cause harmful mutations due to the chemicals in the preservatives, the artificial flavors and the chemically processed cooking involved in its preparation. Having looked at the different categories of edible foods described in Ayurveda, let us now see what the Ayurvedic Principles tell us about-what, how much and when to eat. Why to eat and how to eat.

What to Eat?

The principle of *"Hitbhuk and Ritbhuk"* conveys us that we should always eat properly earned, pure, seasonal and nourishing food. A balanced combination (depending upon the physical and mental labour required in one's daily routine) from the above-described categories of healthy foods would be best suited. For example, you may use wheat, barley, maize, and some pulses, curd, butter, groundnuts, oilseeds, etc, in appropriate quantities with larger amounts of green, leafy and other vegetables; some sprouts should always be part of the food. Don't eat over-cooked or deep fried food; use of spices, salts, sugars and oily substances should be restricted to the essential minimum. Desist consuming toxic substances, stimulating and alcoholic drinks, and non-vegetarian foods.

How Much to Eat?

The answer lies in the principle of *"Mitashi Syat"*. Meaning, eat moderately. Howsoever nourishing or healthy the food may be, it would cause harm if eaten in excess. So, be cautious about the quantity of your diet. Don't fill your tummy more than half its space, leave one-fourth for water and the remaining one-fourth for air. Those doing physical labour need more of proteins, carbohydrates and fats. But those engaged in sedentary and mental work or meditation-devotion etc, should take lighter foods such as boiled vegetables, thin chapatis, milk, sweet fruits, etc.

When to Eat?

As per the vedic routine, one should eat only twice a day after performing *agnihotra* (homam) in the morning and in the evening (before sunset). In today's circumstances, the best timings for the morning meal are any time between 8 a.m. to 12 noon and those for the dinner sometime before 7 p.m. This way the food is easily digested and keeps the body strong and energetic. In any case, be regular in the timings of taking your meals; avoid eating late in the night. One of the major causes of metabolic disorders and varieties of diseases caused thereby is that people keep watching TV and eat very late in the night. Remember! It takes about 8 to11 hours for proper natural digestion of food. Eat only when you feel hungry. Eating is a kind of *agnihotra*. The *ahutis* are made in *agnihotra* only when its fire is lit well; putting the *ahutis* in half-burnt or smoldering wood would only produce smoke instead of healthy effects of *agnihotra*.

Why to Eat?

Eat to maintain and strengthen the health and vigor of your body. Healthy mind resides in a healthy body. The first principle of the *"Yug Nirman Satsankalp"* guided by Gurudev implies - "We shall regard our body as the temple of our soul and maintain its sanctity and health by observing self-restraint and punctuality in our routine". The purpose of food is to sustain healthy and harmonious functioning of the body system, the physical medium of our life, to enable us to perform our duties towards God and His creation. Food is not meant to satiate the greed of our tongue or stomach.

How to Eat?

Take your food gracefully in a calm state of mind, paying full attention to eating; every morsel should be chewed properly. Food should be revered like the *prasada* (offerings made to the Deity). Enough water should be taken before and after the meals. Water is like nectar for our vital functions. Drink at least a tumblerful of water before taking food. Don't drink more than half a bowl of water while eating. Drink sufficient water after about an hour of taking the meals. This helps in proper digestion.

The type of food and mode of eating should also take into account the seasonal effects. The rainy season is very critical with respect to healthcare through controlled food. In this period (known as *visarga* kala in Ayurveda) the sun begins to move towards the winter solstice *(dakshinayana)*. The vata accumulated in the body due to the heat of summer begins to show its ill effects, it diminishes the appetite and causes gastric troubles, etc. Normal digestion also takes longer time in this season because of this vata, which, if one does not take proper care in the selection of food and eating habits, catalyzes the *dosha* of pitta as well. The rise in humidity makes this season risky towards the rise of *kapha dosha*. People prone to cold and cough should therefore be extra careful about their food during the monsoons.

In view of these Ayurvedic observations, one should eat light and easily digestible meals and firmly resist from lavish, heavy stuff. Else the vicious effects of undigested food and associated accumulation and rise of *doshas* will invite one disease after the other, some of which might manifest gradually in the successive seasons. As a preventive measure, drinking water should be boiled in this season and vegetables and salads, etc should also be washed in clean, boiled water. A combination of sweet-sour-salty juicy substance should be used in food to reduce the vata effect. Ginger should be used in food preparations to make it easily digestible. Vegetables like green gourd, lady'sfingers are suitable, as these do not increase gastric problems; use of sprouts or pulses of green-gram and roasted or cooked maize is also beneficial.

Ayurvedic scriptures advise against the use of milk in the month of *shravan* (the second month of rainy season in India) and buttermilk in *bhadon* (the third month of rainy season in India); curd should be generally avoided during the entire season of monsoon. Viral fever, malaria, typhoid, jaundice, conjunctivitis, gastroentritis and skin infections are quite common diseases (in India) during this season. Necessary precautions should be taken in this regard. Preventive herbal medicines may also be used as a support in high-risk areas. (Detailed information and the herbal medicines are available from the Ayruvedic Pharmacy of Shantikunj, Hardwar).

If preventive care is taken as regards taking healthy foods in the rainy season, the winter would prove to be beneficial towards enhancing the vigour and health of the body. Ayurveda also lays stress on spiritual effects of food. We shall present this information extracted from Vedic scriptures.

2

Balancing the Doshas by Food

Lifestyle and diet play important role in balancing doshas. Fortunately, essential oils can help create changes in lifestyle and can be added to the diet. This chapter is intended as a quick reference guide to assist in your day to day living.

REDUCING VATA

Consume warm foods and drinks, oily food, foods with predominately sweet, sour and salty tastes. Oil your body everyday with sesame and essential oils. It is best not to eat alone. Best colors for meditation are yellow, orange, red. Avoid dark colors. Best stones are jade, peridot. Best metal is gold. Avoid cold wind, dampness, excess travel, television, radio, movies, excess talking and thinking. Practice yoga that is calming and grounding. Exercise should be non-vigorous and non-exhaustive, such as tai chi, walking or swimming. Use bulk and toic laxatives like flax seed and psyllium. Avoid diet and fasting, dry foods, cold foods and drinks and foods having predominatly pungent, bitter or astringent tastes. Meals should be small but frequent. It is important to go to bed before 10 p.m. If prone to insomnia, drink teas at night that are calming and soothing. Vata types do better in warm, moist climates. When they live in a cold climate, it is important to protect the head, neck and chest, and keep warm. Use routines to ground, calm and stabilize your life.

REDUCING PITTA

Cool foods and drinks are best; foods with predominately sweet, bitter and astringent tastes. Avoid food with pungent, sour and salty tastes. Have flowers around the house. Bathe in moonlight.

Take walks in the cool air. At night, massage your scalp with coconut oil. Competitive team sports, which promote cooperation are ideal; also activities like hiking which are vigorous and not ego-producing. The best stones, to be carried on the right side of the body, are sapphire, aquamarine, azurite. Take flower baths. Do regular liver flushes; juice of 1 lemon, 1 tablespoon. olive oil, 1 small diced apple or other fruit, blend and drink instead of taking any other item in breakfast (Vata and Kapha may add ginger, garlic and cayenne). Follow diet and avoid restricted foods whenever possible. For meditation colors, use blue and green. Best metal to use on the body is silver. Avoid excessive sauna, hot tub or sunbathing. Seek out what gives you joy.

REDUCING KAPHA

Fast once a week for twenty-four hours. Foods with pungent, bitter and astringent tastes are best. Avoid or reduce sweet, sour and salty foods. No breakfast before 10 a.m., light meal in the evening.Frequent physical and mental exercise; sexual intercourse, minimum sleep. Best colors are yellow, brown and red. Best stones are yellow topaz, coral and diamond. Best metals to use on the body are copper or iron. Take regular baths and saunas to promote sweating.

Note: For any of your problem, you can write to me -

Dr. Rajeev Sharma,

320, Teachers Colony, Bulandshahr (U.P.)

Phone: 05732-221793, 225398,

Email— sharmarajeev108@rediffmail.com,
doctorrajeev108@indiatimes.com

3

Home Treatment by Carrot (Gajar)

Weak Memory

Taking carrot juice with 2 cups of milk (preferably cow's milk) after eating 5-6 almonds early in the moring sharpens memory.

Anaemia

(i) Taking slices of raw carrots and beetroot (chukander) with lemon juice sprinkled on it cures anaemia.

(ii) Taking 250-gms. juice of carrots with spinach juice increases red-blood corpuscles.

Bleeding

Intake of carrots stops Nose bleeding

Applying paste of ground fresh carrot on forehead and above the nostrils stops bleeding from nose. Drinking carrot juice is also advisable.

Headache

Taking juice of carrot, beetroot and cucumber eliminates headache.

Indigestion and Stomach Problems

(i) Taking juice of carrot and spinach after meals cures constipation and helps in easy bowel-movement.

(ii) Taking fresh carrots or its juice regularly cures indigestion, chronic diarrhoea, acidity and other stomach disorders.

(iii) Taking 200 gms. carrot juice mixed with 200 gms. curd (preferably made from goat's milk) in the moming eliminates bleeding and cures amoebiasis.

Cramps

Taking *halwa* of grated red carrots (fried on fire with little *ghee* or butter and mixed with little jaggery) twice a day eliminates cramps and imparts strength.

Rheumatism

(i) Taking carrot juice regularly cures rheumatism.

(ii) or carrot juice mixed with beetroot in equal quantity gives instant relief.

Arthrites

Taking 5 gms. carrot juice with 2½ gms. of juice of kanphool (dandelion) regularly makes the joint supple.

Gout

Taking carrot juice with parsley juice twice a day regularly reduces inflammation of the joints.

Eye Problems

(i) Taking carrot and spinach juice in equal proportion improves eye-sight.

(ii) Taking fresh carrots or its juice daily is very good for eyes and cures even night-blindness.

(iii) Washing eyes with water in which carrots have been boiled gives relief in case of eye-strain.

Asthma

Taking 1 cup of carrot juice mixed with 1 cup of spinach juice regularly thrice a day gives relief in asthma.

Obesity

Taking carrot juice mixed with lettuce juice regularly eliminates extra fat.

Skin Problems

(i) Taking raw carrots or its juice regularly eliminates aches, dryness of the skin, cures itching, removes blood impurities and imparts natural glow.

(ii) Tying heated poultice of carrots on boils cures them.

Eczema

(i) Taking carrot juice 3 times a day cures eczema

(ii) Applying the pulp of carrots on the affected part eliminates the spots left by the disease.

Ringworm

Tying a hot poultice of grated carrot with sendha namak sprinkled on the affected part cures the disease.

Fire-Burn

Applying the crushed pulp of carrot on the affected part and taking its juice eliminates the burning sensation and cures it.

Tonsilitis

Taking carrot juice cures tonsilitis.

Tooth Problems

Taking fresh carrots or 1 cup carrot juice daily strengthens the gums and eliminates all dental problems.

Foul Smell in Mouth

Taking juice of carrots, spinach and cucumber in equal oroportion eliminates foul smell in mouth.

Blood-pressure

Taking carrot juice with spinach juice in 3 : 1 proportion regulates blood pressure.

Urinary Problems

(i) Taking carrot juice regularly twice a day keeps the urinary track clean and unobstructed.

(ii) Taking carrot juice and spinach juice (2 : 1 proportion) eliminates stranguary.

(iii) Taking 2 tsp. ground seeds of carrot boiled in 1 glass of water eliminates stranguary and cures other kidney problems.

Stone

(i) Taking 1 glass of juice of carrot, beetroot, cucumber (in equal proportion) helps in breaking stones and throwing them out.

(ii) Taking carrot juice 3 or 4 times a day is also useful.

(iii) Swallowing ground seeds of carrots with water also helps.

(iv) Taking 1 glass juice of carrot and lettuce (in equal quantity) eliminates stones from gall bladder.

Weak Heart

Taking carrot juice twice a day strengthens the heart.

Liver

Taking 1 cup fresh carrot juice with ½ cup spinach juice everyday cures liver problems. (Gram flour is advised for the patients).

Jaundice

Taking fresh carrot juice or soup or hot decoction of carrots twice a day gives relief in jaundice.

Wound

Tying the pulp of boiled carrots on the wound heals the wounds. Carrot juice should also be taken.

Intestinal Disorders

Taking juice of carrots, cabbage and tomatoes (in equal proportion) daily cures all problems connected with intestines.

Worms

(i) Taking fresh carrot or any preparation of carrot regularly is helpful in expelling worms.

(ii) Taking 1 cup of carrot juice on empty stomach regularly for 10-15 days helps in killing worms and extracting them out of the system.

(iii) Taking 1 glass kanji of carrots regularly for 3-4 weeeks expels the worms.

Pain in Chest

Taking juice of boiled carrots with honey eliminates pain.

Spleen Trouble

Taking pickle of carrots (soak pieces of carrots in water having powder of mustard seeds and little salt for 2 to 3 days) with meals helps in curing spleen troubles.

Diabetes

(i) Taking carrot juice or carrot juice mixed with karela juice daily in the morning helps in secretion of insulin in the body.

(ii) Taking carrot juice with spinach juice (2 :1 proportion) daily is also helpful.

Sexual Weakness

(i) Taking carrot jam with milk two times a day eliminates weakness.

(ii) Taking carrot kheer two times a day is also useful.

Lack of Milk in Breast

(i) Taking black carrots with milk (preferably right from cow's udder) brings enough milk for the child.

(ii) Taking juice of fresh carrots is also advisable.

General Tonic

(i) Eating raw carrot or taking its juice is a good tonic for eyes, skin, physical and mental -development.

(ii) Giving 2-3 tablespoon. carrot juice to weak children makes them physically strong.

4

Home Treatment by Radish

Constipation

Taking fresh leaves of radish with kala namak cures constipation.

Indigestion and Stomach Problems

(i) Taking fresh radish with or without carrots and tomatoes eliminates acidity.

(ii) Taking radish with sendha namak and black pepper sprinkled on it at meal time improves digestion and eliminates wind and acidity.

(iii) Taking juice of fresh radish, cabbage and tomato cures flatulence.

(iv) Taking juice of fresh radishwith little sendha namak twice a day cures stomach-ache and other problems of digestion.

(v) Taking the raw roots of radish helps in digestion and increases appetite.

(vi) Taking radish pieces (soaked for two days in mustard seeds powder) brings back appetite.

Urinary problems

(i) Taking 30-40 gms of fresh radish juice eliminates irritation and pain while urinating and also cures stranguary.

(ii) Taking fresh leaves juice twice or thrice a day or juice of root of fresh radish is also useful.

Stones

(i) Taking 1 cup juice of radish 3 or 4 times a day and chewing its fresh leaves or taking Radish seeds water (35 gms seeds, which are inside the covering of the beans of radish, boiled in half litre water till it is reduced to half for few days helps in breaking stones and throwing them out.

(ii) Taking juice of fresh Radish elps in stopping the formation of gallstones.

Hoarse Throat

(i) Taking about 4-5 gms of ground seeds of Radish with lukewarm water-clears the throat.

(ii) Gargling with lukewarm radish water also helps.

Mouth-Blisters

Gargling with radish juice mixed with water in the same proportion and little salt cures it.

Foul Breath

Taking radish juice with mishri eliminates foul breath.

Lethargy

Taking pieces of white radish and its soft leaves with lemon juice sprinkled on it eliminates lethargy.

Hiccough

Chewing soft leaves of 3-4 radish cures hiccough.

Ringworm

Applying heated paste of seeds of radish ground in lemon-juice on the affected part is useful in curing it.

Eczema, Itching and Other Skin Problems

(i) Applying paste of freshly ground radish pulp for 1 hour before taking bath is helpful in curing eczema.

(ii) Taking radish with salad in meals with lemon juice sprinkled on it removes blood impurities and cures itching.

(iii) Applying ground pulp of Radish on the face till it gets dried up before washing with cold water cures acnes on face.

(iv) Taking one radish alongwith leaves or its juice regularly and applying the ground pulp on face eliminates black spots and freckles.

(v) Massaging with radish juice eliminates wrinkles.

Jaundice

Taking fresh raw radish or Radish juice with sugar or Radish juice and sugarcane juice early in the morning cures jaundice.

Worms

Taking radish juice with little sendha namak and lemon juice after meals destroys worms and throws them out.

Arthritis

(i) Taking fomentation of steam of hot water of radish soft leaves (boiled first in a closed utensil) eliminates swelling and pain.

(ii) Taking 1 tabelspoon ground seeds of Radish with water is also useful.

(iii) Taking juice of radish with sugar is useful.

Menstrual Problems

(i) Taking 2-3 gms of ground seeds of radish 3-times a day regulates and relieves pain during menses.

(ii) Taking fresh leaves of radish cures pimples due to lack of bleeding in menses.

Fire-Burns

Applying paste of ground Radish pulp on the burnt portion helps in quick healing.

Eye-Care

Taking one radish a day is very good for eye-sight.

Whooping Cough

Taking juice of radish with sugar-cane juice in equal quantity and little ginger juice gives relief in this.

Insect-bite

(i) Applying juice of radish or slice of radish with salt (to be changed after 5 minutes) on the affected part eliminates poisonous effect of scorpion.

(ii) Taking radish juice after 3 or 4 hours relieves the affect of poison.

Piles

(i) Taking fresh radish or 1 cup of juice with 1 tsp pure *ghee* twice a day helps in curing it.

(ii) Taking slices of radish (kept in open with salt sprinkled on it overnight) empty stomach in the morning,.

(iii) Taking slices of radish fried in ghee is also very useful.

Sexual weakness

(i) Taking radish regularly helps in getting back lost sexual power.

(ii) Taking 2 gms of powder of seeds of radish (dry 50 gms seeds of Radish powder and them Strain) with butter or cream regularly for atleast 8-10 days eliminates sexual weakness.

5

Home Treatment by Ginger (Adrak)

Ginger grows best in tropical and sub tropical areas, which have good rainfall with hot and humid conditions during the summer. This member of the *Zingiberaceae* family originated in Southeast Asia and has been introduced to many parts of the globe where it proliferates in suitable environments.

Belief in the medicinal properties of ginger existed in ancient Indian and oriental cultures where ginger was used alone or as a component in herbal remedies.

This practice continues today in many areas of the world, including Africa, Brazil, China, Fiji, Indonesia, Mexico, Peru, Sudan and Thailand. Ginger was introduced to Europe and other areas by Dutch, Portuguese, Arab and Spanish explorers or traders from around the 13th to 16th centuries.

The rhizome or "root" is the part of the plant that is harvested and is found entirely under the surface of the soil. The vast majority of the harvested ginger is consumed fresh or in dehydrated form, while some commercial ginger is preserved. In Australia, ginger for sugar preserving is harvested after five months before fibre content reaches a level that affects eating quality. Drying of ginger commences after seven months for manufacture of dried whole root and ginger powder.

In recent times there has been scientific research undertaken to test out the validity of the medicinal claims made about ginger. A study of the research shows that there have been some exciting results with respect to the medicinal properties of ginger including, anti-emetic effect or control of nausea and vomiting, prevention of coronary artery disease, healing and prevention of both arthritic conditions and stomach ulcers. In addition, ginger has been shown to be effective against tumor growth, rheumatism, migraine and is active as an antioxidant in the body.

One of the most detailed literature studies on ginger and its medicinal properties is found in Research Herbalist Paul Schulick`s book *"Common Spice or Wonder Drug? Ginger"* (1993, Herbal Free Press, Brattleboro, Vermont, USA). This book is recommended to any person interested in exploring the uses of ginger as a natural remedy and maintainer of good health. His work links early herbalists claims with modern scientific research and lists over 300 references.

CURATIVE PROPERTIES

Anti-emetic and Anti-motion Sickness

Powdered ginger root has been compared to standard drugs used in combating postoperative nausea and vomiting. Tests have shown that the requirement for postoperative antiemetics was lower in those patients receiving ginger. Ginger is "an effective and promising prophylactic antiemetic, which may be especially useful for day case surgery.

It has been reported that ginger was effective in reducing postoperative nausea and vomiting in a group of 60 women after major gynecological surgery. "There were statistically significantly fewer recorded incidences of nausea in the group that received ginger root compared to the placebo.

Patients who undergo photopheresis suffer nausea due to the untake of 8-MOP durg which is required during the treatment. In a controlled trial, it has been shown that the ingestion of ginger prior to 8-MOP, may substantially reduce the nausea effect.

The possibility of side effects such as gastric emptying after taking ginger as an antiemetic has been investigated. When 16 healthy volunteers were allocated 1 g of ginger or placebo randomly in a double-blind crossover trial, it was found that ginger ingestion had no effect on gastric emptying. It was reported that, "The antiemetic effect of ginger is not associated with an effect on gastric emptying". No adverse effects were noted.

One of the most famous reports on the effects of ginger on motion sickness was reported in the British medical journal *The Lancet*.

In this clinical trial, 39 men and women who reported "very high susceptibility to motion sickness" were tested. Motion sickness was induced by being subjected to a rotating, tilted chair while blindfolded under controlled conditions. It was found that ginger was significantly more effective in reducing motion sickness than the antihistamine dimenhydrinate and a placebo.

A Danish controlled trial on the open sea involved 80 naval cadets who were "unaccustomed to sailing in heavy seas". It was reported that "ginger root reduced the tendency to vomiting and cold sweating significantly better than the placebo did".

Pharmacological studies of the antimotion actions of ginger would indicate that ginger is effective in controlling motion sickness by the direct action of ginger's active components on the gastric system.

Anti-Inflammatory (Rheumatism)

More than 200 potential drugs have been tested through the 1990s in order to find a cure for rheumatism and musculo skeletal ailments. These have included non-steroidal anti-inflammatory drugs, corticosteroids, gold salts, disease modifying anti-rheumatic drugs, methotrexate and cyclosporine. None of these have found to be safe.

A Danish study has found that ginger ingestion is significant in relieving pain associated with rheumatoid arthritis, osteoarthritis and muscular disorder patients.

In this study 56 patients (28 rheumatoid, 18 osteo, 10 muscular) were studied over periods ranging from 3 months to 2.5 years. Three quarters of the 56 arthritis patients experienced, "to varying degrees, relief in pain and swelling." All of the muscular discomfort patients experienced, "relief in pain." Over the period of the testing, no patients reported any adverse effects from consistent ginger consumption. Other studies have produced similar results, where patients reported that ginger "produced better relief of pain, swelling and stiffness than the administration of non-steroidal anti-inflammatory drugs".

Gingerols found in ginger, have been identified as active compounds which are potent inhibitors of the biosynthesis of prostaglandins, which, in an oversupply situation will cause inflammation.

Anti Ulcer

A common side effect of treating inflammation with modern drugs is that ulcers in the digestive system can be created or their condition made worse. Ginger can not only relieve the symptoms of inflammation, it also protects the creation of digestive ulcers. Paul Schulick states, "Whatever advantage non-steroidal anti-inflammatory drugs have in the strength of their anti-inflammatory or thermoregulatory effects, ginger compensates for it with an absence of side effects and alternative effects."

Extensive laboratory testing, often involving the use of rats, has brought about the identification of six anti-ulcer compounds contained in ginger.

Ginger and the Circulatory System

Ginger has been found to be beneficial in reducing platelet aggregation which leads to coronary artery disease, while having no effect on blood lipids or blood sugar. Healthy people, patients with C.A.D.(coronary artery disease) and non-insulin dependent diabetes sufferers were all the subjects of an Indian study which found that a 10g single dose of powdered ginger,"significantly reduced platelet aggregation" in C.A.D. patients.

Rats have been clinically studied with the introduction of ginger after having their cholesterol levels artificially increased. Researchers state," Inclusion of 1% cholesterol in the diet of rats increased serum cholesterol levels significantly, but addition of fresh ginger together with the cholesterol significantly reduced this increase. Ginger was shown to be antihypercholesterolaemic." It has also been reported that ginger inhibits the biosynthesis of cholesterol in rat liver.

Paul Shulick makes the point, "that literally hundreds of thousands of lives can be saved and emphasizes that ginger should be in everyone's daily supplement routine.

Antioxidant

Ginger contains antioxidant properties that even outperform commonly used chemical antioxidants. Ginger is rated in a number of studies to possess a free radical-inhibiting index even greater than that of commercial antioxidant preservatives BHA and BHT.

Ginger has been found to inhibit lipid peroxidation in rat liver microcosms and successfully scavenge superoxide anions.In an American study 21 compounds (including gingerol related compounds) were isolated from ginger. It was found that "most of the isolated compounds exhibited stronger antioxidative effect than alpha-tocopherol"(vitamin E).

The antioxidant powers of ginger have been proven in applications where ginger extract was added to meat products. "The antioxodative effectiveness of ginger extract was further tested with fresh, frozen and precooked pork patties. The shelf life of all products determined by TBA value was improved by the inclusion of ginger extract.

Other Properties of Ginger

Researchers have found that extracts of ginger possess anti-skin tumor effects when placed directly on the skin of mice. In addition it has been found that gingerol from ginger inhibits the tumor promoter Epstein-Barr virus (EBV) activation.

Ginger treatments have been found to be useful in treatment of migraine, where it is proposed that pain relief from ginger may occur without any of the side effects that occur with standard treatments. Ginger has also been successfully trialled in tests with 30 women who were suffering from hyperemesis gravidarum,which is a severe nausea, which can complicate a large proportion of pregnancies. After the trial it was found that relief was "significantly greater" with oral ginger powder capsule treatment.

Ginger has been shown to be effective against the growth of both Gram-positive and Gram-negative bacteria including Escherichia Coli, Proteus vulgaris, Salmonella typhimurium, Staphylococcus aureus and Streptococcus viridans. A 1990 Japanese study showed that the gingerol and shogaol components of ginger could kill Anisakis larvae. Anisakis being one of the principle parasites which find hosts in millions of people around the globe.

In addition to the previously mentioned antiemetic properties of ginger there are many other benefits associated with the digestive system. Chinese medicine has incorporated ginger in remedies for the digestive system for centuries and it is regularly used as a calmative for stomach upsets. Other digestive benefits from ginger are the natural enzyme action on protein digestion, stimulation of digestion, pro-biotic support of the natural gut flora, anti-diarreal properties and liver protection.

6

Home Treatment by Onion (Pyaz)

Onion is a source of energy and acts as a stimulant, increases vigour and vitality, acts as an expectorant and diuretic, slows the heart beat, prevents flatulence and dyspepsia. It is useful in various diseases.

Cough

Onion juice mixed with ginger juice and honey act as an expectorant.

Cold

Eating raw onion or applying onion juice on the forehead helps in controlling cold.

Asthma

Onion juice mixed with ginger juice, black pepper and salt or ground onion with honey helps in controlling asthma and problems of throat, tonsils and lungs.

Tuberclosis

Intake of raw onion prevents and guards the attack of T B. germs and also helps in eradicating TB.

Pain in Ears

2 to 3 drops of lukewarm onion juice cures the pain in ears.

Eyes

One drop of onion diluted with rose water helps in improving the eyesight and eliminates eye ailments.

Hysteria

Unconsciousness due to hysteria is cured by making the patient smell onion or by rubbing his feet with crushed onion.

Cholera

(i) One cup of onion juice mixed with juice of one lemon, one teaspoon of ginger juice, pinch of salt (table salt or kaala namak) given in four equal doses in a day prevents cholera.

(ii) One teaspoon of onion juice with little salt given two hourly or one spoon of onion juice mixed with juice of mint leaves given every hour helps in cholera.

Jaundice

Small onion cut into four pieces soaked in vinegar or lemon-juice taken with salt and black pepper twice a day helps in curing jaundice.

Urinary Problems

Onion juice taken in hot water acts as diuretic.

Stone (Pathari)

Onion juice mixed with sugar (sharbat) helps in breaking the stone.

Diarrhoea

Applying paste of onion on navel region helps in curing diarrhoea.

Blood from the Nose

Few drops of onion juice put in the nose helps in stopping bleeding from the nose.

Skin-diseases

(i) Onion mixed with turmeric powder and mustard oil, heated on fire into a paste and applied on bowl and abscess, helps in draining out pus.

(ii) One-fourth cup of onion-juice mixed with one cup of water used for washing the wounds and bowls etc. and applying a dressing of the same acts as a disinfectant and removes itching.

Heat-Stroke

(i) In summer eating of raw-onion prevents heat stroke.

(ii) Applying the onion paste on the feet counteracts the effect of heatstroke.

Intoxication

Onion juice reduces the effect of over-intoxication.

Menstrual Disorders

Onion made into a curry with condiments or onion juice mixed with gur taken regularly helps in curing menstural disorders.

Acne

(i) Applying onion-juice on acnes cures the overgrowth (massa).

(ii) Seeds of onion ground and mixed with milk beautifies the skin by cleansing the spots etc.

(iii) Rubbing paste of onion with lime helps in removing the small overgrowth of skin.

Insect-bite

Applying paste of onion helps in curing the poisonous effect of bite of insects like honey-bee, yellow jacket, scorpion etc.

Baldness

Rubbing onion juice on the bald area of the head helps in new growth.

Dental Problems

Eating raw-onion prevents bacterial growth in the mouth, stops dental decay, helps in curing dental problems.

Insomnia

One teaspoon of onion juice mixed with milk or honey taken at bed-time induces sleep.

Arthritis

Rubbing of onion juice with oil of sesamum cures arthritis. Besides medicinal properties onion has other uses also.

Keeping of onion piece in the room is helpful to remove the smell of fresh paint in the room.

Keeping one onion in pocket is advised for preventing heat-stroke.

Tying of a piece of onion near the light dispels mosquitos, insects etc. coming in the room.

Keeping white onion prevents snakes from entering the house.

7

Home Treatment by Garlic (Garlic)

Garlic is a gastric stimulant and helps in digestion, acts as an anti-flatulant, carminative and diaphoretic. It is stimulant of kidneys and skin and is diuretic in nature. It is a tonic giving strength and vitality, an expectorant having a special effect on the bronchial and pulmonary secretions, beneficial for eyes and brain and helps in healing fractured bones and is a great antiseptic. It has Allicin which has the property to destroy even those germs which are not killed by *Penicillin*. It is thus a very powerful germicidal.

Heart Problems

(i) As diluting agent for blood—regular eating of garlic and then having milk boiled in it controls assimilation of cholestrol.

(ii) Chewing 4 or 5 cloves of garlic—given at the time of heart attack prevents heart failure and advised till medical aid is procured.

Paralysis

(i) 25 grams ground garlic cloves boiled in milk—till it becomes thick (like Kheer) to be taken when cooled in the morning for atleast a month.

Also massage the body with oil. (Boil 250 gms ground garlic sheliots with 500 gms mustard oil in an iron till it is burnt. Put some camphor in it. Cool it and keep it in bottle for massage).

(ii) Eating 7 ground garlic cloves with one tsp of fresh butter also helps in curing paralysis.

High Blood pressure

Taking six drops of garlic juice with fresh water regularly reduces hypertension.

Bronchitis

Paste of garlic with onion applied on the chest as poultice cures bronchitis.

Bile, Cough, Wind

For bile—use of ground garlic with sugar; for cough with honey (especially in winter and spring) and for wind with ghee (especially in rainy season) is highly recommended.

Asthma

(i) Garlic juice taken with hot water twice a day.

(ii) One dried clove with little salt twice a day.

(iii) 10 drops of garlic juice with 2 teaspoon of honey cures Asthma. It can be administered at the time of attack also.

Tuberclosis

Pulmonary infections including TB is controlled by:

(i) Regular intake of garlic because its rich contents of sulphuric acid, destroys TB germs.

(ii) Chewing 10 cloves of garlic boiled in 250 gm. milk and then having that milk helps in curing TB.

(iii) Chewing of 3-4 cloves of garlic 3 times a day reduces cough, increases appetite, Induces sleep and helps in curing TB of lungs.

(iv) Smelling cotton-wool soaked in garlic juice carries its strong smell to lungs which helps in destroying all germs.

Whooping Cough, Cold and Cough

(i) Regular intake of 3-5 cloves of garlic cures cold and cough.

(ii) 6-7 drops of garlic juice mixed with sharbat of pomegranate cures all types of cold and cough and even whooping cough.

(iii) Taking a cloves of garlic with 5 soaked, peeled and ground almonds and mishri in the morning taken for 3-4 days cures whooping cough.

(iv) 8-10 drops of garlic juice mixed with 4 gms of honey 4 times a day cures whooping cough.

(v) Making the child wear a mala (garland) having 2 cloves of garlic helps in curing whooping cough.

(vi) 5 drops of garlic in hot water given 2 or 3 times a day cures frequent and violent coughing spells.

Sore Throat

Gargles with hot water with few drops of galic juice cures sore throat.

Sneezing

Juice of 5 to 7 cloves of garlic with hot water taken once stops frequent sneezing.

Malaria

Application of garlic juice on nails of hands and feet before fever and taking 1 tsp garlic juice with 1 tsp fresh water thrice a day cures malaria.

Jaundice

4 ground cloves of garlic mixed with half cup hot milk for 4-5 days helps in curing jaundice.

Night discharge

Chewing 1-2 cloves of garlic with 1 cup hot milk before bedtime stops night discharge.

Migraine

Paste of garlic applied on forehead or near the ears for 3-4 minutes and putting 2 drops of garlic juice in the nostril (of the affected side) relieves pain of migraine.

Ear-ache

Drop of garlic juice boiled in little mustard oil relieves ear-ache.

Pain in Arms

Fried ground garlic and sonth in ghee mixed with honey be kept in bottle. Taking 10 gms of this and drinking hot milk, tea or coffee in winters relieves pain.

Impotency

Keep 200 gms ground garlic mixed with 600 gm. pure honey in a bottle in a sack of wheat for 21 or 31 days.

(i) Taking 10 gms of that paste-followed by drinking lukewarm milk early in the morning for 21 or 31 days gives extraordinary strength and helps in curing impotency.

(ii) Chewing 4 cloves of garlic slowly early in the morning followed by drinking lukewarm taking ghee regularly in winters gives extraordinary strength to men. It removes infertility in women.

Arthrities

(i) Massage the body with garlic oil (250 gms. ground cloves of garlic boiled in 500 gm mustard oil and in burnt in an iron karahi).

(ii) Take pieces of 3 or 4 cloves of garlic boiled in milk or kheer made of ground 3 or 4 cloves in milk before going to bed.

This has to be taken regularly with gradual increase in quantity for 6 weeks or more to cure arthirities.

Gastric Ulcer and Acidity

After 2 or 3 sips of water taking ground cloves of garlic and after meals and drinking little water cures gastric ulcer, hypertension and other ailments due to atmospheric and water-pollution. Eating cloves of garlic checks excessive acidity.

Diarrhoea

Taking 2 or 3 cloves of garlic with water has a soothing effect on varied types of diarrhoea.

Flatulence, Sciatica

Small dose of decoction (strain after boiling together 6 ounces of garlic with 2 pints of water and 4 pints of milk till the water is evaporated) given regularly cures flatulence, sciatica.

Round Worms

Intake of a cloves of galic for sometime acts as a vermifuge in expelling round-worms.

Frost-bite, Leucoderma, Ringworm, Alopecia

Apart from eating raw garlic-local application of garlic paste on affected part for 2 to 4 minutes is advisable.

Itching

Massaging the body with garlic oil purifies blood and cures itching.

Urinary problems

Paste of garlic applied below navel relieves strangury.

Infantile Convulsions

Poultice of garlic applied to the spine is recommended.

Pyorrhoea

(i) Regularly taking 6-10 drops of garlic in 1 tsp. of honey cures pyorrhoea.

(ii) Boil garlic in mustard oil. When garlic gets fried—strain the oil, cool it and mix it with fried ground 30 gm. Ajwayan and 15 gm. sendha salt.

Brushing the teeth with this cures bad breath and pyorrhoea. It is to be done for 2-3 months.

Baldness

Applying garlic juice on the bald head and leaving it to dry 3 times a day for few weeks helps in hair-growth.

Bites of Venomous Reptiles and Dogs

(i) Paste of garlic applied on the bites of venomous reptiles counteracts poison.

(ii) 5-7 ground shellots of garlic mixed with 1 pint of milk adminstered immediately after bite counteracts the poison.

Hysteria

Inhaling the smell of cloves of garlic kept near the nostrils helps to recover from swooning.

Antiseptic for cleaning Wounds

Mixture of garlic juice and water is very effective antiseptic lotion for cleaning all types of wounds etc.

Garlic is scientifically admitted and proved to be very useful and good for health. It can be classified as a therapeutic food used raw or in cooking. Because of its medicinal properties, it is a panacea for a number of ailments. It is rightly called 'King of Herbs' easily available to rich and poor alike.

Some people, however, disapprove of garlic because of its strong odour. To prevent or suppress odour of Lahsun the following may be noted:

(i) Chewing roasted coffee grains, fresh parsley leaves, cardamom seeds, fresh coriander leaves, washing out the mouth with lemon juice, eating apples diminishes the odour of garlic.

(ii) Lemon juice or vinegar put in garlic juice suppresses its odour. Smell of garlic from hands can be removed by sprinkling the hands with salt and cleaning them properly with cold water.

Precautions

(i) In large doses it is an irritant and produces flatulence, headache, nausea, vomitting etc. So it should be taken in limited quantity.

(ii) As a local stimulant and irritant, it reddens the skin and causes Vesication. So its application should not be for more than 2-3 minutes.

(iii) Not admissible for pregnant woman.

8

Home Treatment by Lemon (Lebu/Nimbu)

Botanically it is called citrus acid. It is a small tree or spreading bush of the rue family (Rutaceae). The lemon forms a spreading bush or a small tree 10 to 20 feet high if not trained or pruned. Its young leaves have a decidedly reddish tint; later they turn green. In some varieties; the young leaves of the lemon are angular; some have sharp thorns at the axilae of the leaves. The flowers with a sweet odour are rather large, solitary or in small clusters in the axilae of the leaves. Reddish tinted in the bud, the petalis are white above and reddish purple below.

General Information

The fruit is oval with a broad low apical nipple and having 8 to 10 segments. The outer rind or peel is yellow when ripe and rather thick in some varieties is prominently glandular dotted. The white spongy inner part of the peel called the mesocarp is nearly tasteless and is the chief source of commercial grades of pectin. The seeds are small, ovoid, pointed, sometimes few or more. The pulp is decidedly acid. Young lemon starts bearing fruits as early as the third year after planting and commercial crop may be expected during the fifth year. The average orchard yield per tree is 1500 lemons a year.

The humble lemon contains most of the vitamins and minerals. It has magical and wonderful healing powers. It is a citrus fruit. Other citrus fruits are orange, mandarine, tangerine, narangi, musumbi (lime), grape-fruit, grape, and shaddock. All citrus fruits are very rich sources of vitamins A, B and C. They also contain appreciable amounts of iron and calcium.

Rich Source of Vitamin C

Vitamin C in the diet helps the body to grow and maintain collagen. They explain that collagen is a gelatin like gristle that holds billions of cells together in the body. It is found in ligaments, joints, bones, gum tissues and in the walls of all the blood vessels. It also gives elasticity and strength to the connective tissue. Again vitamin C is necessary to the normally healing rate of wounds and to prevent bruises from discolouring the skin for too long time. Its function is also to strengthen the body's resistance to infection and maintain tissue integrity of teeth, bones and gums.

Vitamin C in adequate quantity must be taken daily and if its deficiency is continued over a long period of time, the gums may become tender and bleed easily, joints may hurt and swell, black and blue marks may appear readily at the slightest bruise, the chance of haemorrhage which may result from a 'stroke' is far greater and colds may be taken frequently. Deficiency of vitamin C may cause scurvy. Therefore vitamin C is absolutely necessary to fortify the body against infections and cold.

Daily requirement of Vitamin C

Men	—	75 mg
Women	—	70 mg
Lactating women	—	150 mg
Pregnant women	—	100 mg
Children:		
Infants	—	30 mg
1 to 3 yrs.	—	35 mg
4 to 6 yrs.	—	50 mg
7 to 9 yrs.	—	60 mg
Boys:		
10 to 12 yrs.	—	75 mg
13 to 15 yrs.	—	80 mg
16 to 20 yrs.	—	100 mg

Girls:

10 to 12 yrs.	—	75 mg
13 to 15 yrs.	—	80 mg
16 to 20 yrs.	—	80 mg

Fruits containing Vitamin C

Whole orange	—	75 mg
4 oz orange juice	—	50 mg
Large grape fruit	—	150 mg
Medium size tangerine	—	25 mg
Lemon juice 1 tbs	—	7 mg
Lime (musumbi)	—	75 mg

Where extra vitamin C is needed

Smoking and alcoholic beverages: It is found on research that smoking causes great damage to vitamin C content in the human body. One cigarette destroys 25 mg of vitamin C in the body which means that 500 mg is neutralised for every packet of cigarettes smoked. If smoking is continued throughout the morning, the store of vitamin C will be entirely neutralised. To replace, foods containing vitamin C (ascorbic acid) must be taken during lunch, although this replacement will also be depleted if one continues to smoke in the afternoon. So a habitual smoker will always require much more vitamin C than the non-smoker. This will explain why those who smoke are more prone to infections than those who do not.

Stress, strain and fatigue: Stress disorders demand increased intake of vitamin C. It is found that more than fifty common disorders are attributed to stress and strain.

Diseases and injuries: Patients suffering from burns or injuries require increased intake of vitamin C which is necessary for tissue regeneration. The use of antibiotics or barbiturates also causes deficiency of vitamin C in the body. So citrus fruits must be consumed in adequate quantities daily in order to keep healthy.

Old Age (Aging): Older people require more vitamin C than younger people. It is found that large quantities of vitamin C strengthen the capillaries in certain vascular diseases like diabetes. Citrus fruits as a source of vitamin C and other nutrients are particularly important food for persons whose normal digestive functions have been disturbed by illness or advanced age. The high vitamin C content of citrus fruits not only tends to restore normalcy but militates against further infection and helps to heal tissue and capillary lesions.

A senile person is forgetful, confused and his speech rambles. He repeats a question that has been just answered. Memory is so poor that the individual does not recognise members of his own family. So senile patients and those approaching old age need substantial quantities of vitamin C to protect their brain from damage and to fight infections.

Ascorbic acid alone may be used in the preservation of vitamin C and treatment for deficiency, but the natural juice of citrus fruits will be more efficient and more complete in their action. In the citrus fruits, ascorbic acid is always accompanied by a bonus of other vital nutrients which nature in her wisdom has supplied. But the citrus fruits or juices should be taken fresh.

Nutritional Value of Citrus Fruits

Citrus fruits are rich in vitamin C and also contain numerous other vitamin, especially A, inositol and vitamin B complex. They also supply appreciable supplementary amounts of minerals with which it becomes easy to maintain health properly. Minerals build rich blood, strong bones, nerve tissues and assist in regulating the body. Calcium found in orange makes them a valuable food for infants as it is necessary for growing bodies. Oranges are also useful for older people.

Lemons as Medicine

Lemon juice cures menorrhagia, nose-bleeding, hepatitis, gastric ulcer if taken several times daily. Of all foods which have also been used as medicines, lemons are the most commonly known. The custom of using a slice of lemon when eating a fish dinner was originally intended for remedial purposes rather than for flavouring.

It was believed that if a fish bone were to be accidentally swallowed during the meals, the juice of lemon could dissolve it. Lemons have been used as a household remedy for colds, rheumatism, sore throat, gastric and liver troubles, headache, heartburn, biliousness etc. Lemon juice mixed with glycerine is used for chapped lips or chilblains. For constipation, the juice of a lemon is taken in a glass of hot water half an hour before breakfast. Local application of lemon juice is used to allay irritation caused by bites of gnats and similar insects.

Dr. Fred R. Klenner has described most elaborately the various uses of lemon in his book *'The Key to Good Health: Vitamin C'*. Lemon juice is very useful in arthritis, cold, hypertension, sun-stroke and menorrhagia.

LEMON JUICE IN DISEASES

Arthritis, Rheumatic Diseases

A few drinks of lemon juice is the surest remedy for rheumatic fever, painful joints, lumbago and sciatica. There will be no cardiac complications. Those with incipient arthritis were given ascorbic acid therapy and similar results were achieved.

Common Cold

Lemon juice or vitamin C tablets taken three or four times daily along with garlic cures cough and cold.

Oedema

Oedema of the muscular region produced by vascular decompensation often responds more rapidly when 10 to 33 ounces of orange or grape-fruit juice is given in addition to 500 mg of vitamin C for three or four days.

Hypertension, and Cardiovascualr Diseases in the Aged

Many illnesses of the aged may be prevented with an adequate intake of vitamin C daily. Particularly cerebrovascular diseases and heart disorders may be largely reduced.

Prickly Heart

Quick relief is obtained by taking a few drops of lemon juice daily.

Shock

To prevent surgical shock surgeons apply ascorbic acid routinely before and after surgery. 500 mg by mouth one hour before surgery to patients of average weight helps to combat traumatic shock. Vitamin C is extremely useful in preventing shock and post-operative weakness.

Menorrhagia and Haemorrhage

A few drinks of lemon juice or narangi juice will certainly give some relief in acute menorrhagia.

Asthma

Many cases of asthma have been relieved by taking a half-spoonful of lemon-juice before each meal and upon retiring.

Cough and Cold

Roasted lemon when properly prepared is one of the most effective remedies for cough and cold.

Corns

Lemon juice applied to corns a few times a day makes an effective remedy. Bind the corn and leave it overnight, you can expect wonderful results.

Headache

Lemon tea relieves headache.

Heartburn

One glass of lemon juice, gives relief from heartburn.

Nausea, Vomiting and Travel Sickness

If one takes a glass of lemon juice before leaving home, one can return from travelling without any trouble.

Sun-Stroke or Heat-Stroke

Lemon or lime (musumbi) juice prevents sun-stroke or heat-stroke.

Whooping Cough

Lemon or musumbi (lime) juice is a household remedy for whooping cough.

Weakness and General Debility

Lemon or musumbi (lime) juice offers an excellent remedy in general debility and weakness.

Low Vitality

Lemon or lime (musumbi) juice removes this condition very quickly.

Removing Stains

Use clear lemon juice; it will remove stains from the hands.

Hair Tonic and Teeth Cleaner

Dr. Donald Law in his book *'Herbs for cooking and for healing'* has said that there are over 20 varieties of lemon but the juice of all of them is most helpful as a remedy for purifying the blood, for rubbing into the scalp against falling hair. Lemon juice mixed with shampoo acts as a tonic to the scalp. From medieval times the skin of lemon has been chewed to act as a cleaner of teeth and strengthener of gums. Naturopaths frequently recommend a course of lemon juice and water to rid the body of accumulated poisons and debris. For extracting more juice from a lemon place it in an oven for a few minutes and bake it slowly. The humble lemon contains vitamin A, B, C, G and the rare vitamin P.

Carbuncle, Abscess, Dysentery, Jaundice

Lemon juice cures erysipelas, carbuncle and abscess. Dysentery quickly disappears after a few drinks of pure lemon or musumbi juice. Some naturopaths also cured diabetes by giving pure lemon or musumbi juice to drink. Jaundice and clotting of arteries by cholesterol are alleviated by prolonged course of lemon juice. Many diseases of the respiratory system can be cured by including lemon juice in the diet. It may be sweetened by adding sugar to it.

Scurvy

Dr. Richard Lucas in his book *'Nature's Medicines'* has expressed the view that lemons were highly valued in ancient times as medicine and for prevention of scurvy. Scurvy is a disease characterised by a spongy condition of the gums, loosening of the teeth, foul breath, debility and anaemia. There is also a tendency to haemorrhage especially into the mucous membranes and skin. Scurvy was common among the crewmen on the old time sailing vessels where the diet consisted entirely of dried or salted biscuits or loaf. The scientific answer to scurvy is vitamin C which is available in plenty in citrus fruits.

Dr. Wood and Ruddock in their book *'Encyclopaedia of health and home'* remarked that lemon juice may be used in curing asthma, cough and cold, corns, headache, heartburn, vomiting and whooping cough.

Blackheads

Dr. M. Grieve in his book *'Modern Herbal'* has said that washing the face with lemon juice and water is said to remove tan, freckles or blackheads.

Dandruff

Lemon juice rubbed in the scalp before shampooing is considered an effective remedy for dandruff. A lemon milk preparation is employed for whitening and softening the skin of the hands and face. Lemon juice is an all-round beauty aid. Lemon juice makes a nice rinse for the hair. It will remove the soap film much better than plain water.

Other Uses

Dr. Joseph E. Meyer in his book *'Nature's Remedies'* has said that a few drops of lemon juice sprinkled over sliced bananas, apples or grapes will prevent them from turning brown for a considerable period of time. Frequent applications of lemon juice is said to remove ink, rust, or mild stains from cloth. For this purpose some recipes call for the addition of milk or salt to lemon juice.

Dr. A.N. Ghei in his book on *'The Book of Food and Nutrition'* has expressed that the additin of lemon juice to rice, boiled fish etc. gives a special flavour and has some specific action in promoting digestion. It is also used in salads. Being very rich in vitamin C, it acts as an antiscorbutic.

Dr. W. Hale White in his book *'Material Medica'* has said that lemon-juice is used to relieve thirst and to make effervescing mixtures and drinks. Its action is the same as that of citric acid.

Nicholas Culpepper in his book *'Complete Herbal'* has written that fruit and vegetable juice offers an excellent remedy for arthritis, bronchitis, intestinal disorders, stomach disoders and urinary disorders. He has observed that cooking destroys most of the natural vitamins and minerals. He has advised to consume raw fresh fruit and vegetable juice as far as practicable.

Harrison Dayal in his book *'Ancient Indian Energy Food'* and Kristine Nolfi in her book *'My experiences with living food'* have given various uses of lemon. Roman Bernard in his book *'Herbal elixirs of life'* has identified lemon as the 'miracle fruit'. Nelson Coon in his book *'Using plants for healing'* has narrated the various medicinal uses of lemon.

9

Home Treatment by Emblic Myrobalan (Amla)

Hindus consider amla tree as very sacred. It is believed that having foot under amla tree on 'Akshya Navami' in month of Kartika-leads to happiness and prosperity.

Amla is unique in this that-the fruit does not leave its chemical ingredients even when heated on fire. Every single part of the fruit—rind, pulp, seed etc is used for medicinal purposes. Moreover, Amla tree purifies the air and atmosphere.

Amla is sour and bitter in taste. It controls imbalances caused by va (wind), pitta (bile) and kaph (phlegm.), and is very effective in controlling digestive problems. It strengthens cardiac muscles, invigorates physic and mental faculties, improves eyesight, imparts natural glow and lustre in the body and hair. It is very useful in diarrhoea and is diuretic in nature. Its regular intake leads to healthy long life.

General Tonic

(i) Taking one raw amla everyday in the morning removes general weakness of the different parts of the body.

(ii) Taking milk in the morning after licking one teaspoon of ground amla powder mixed with honey imparts freshness and strength to the body.

(iii) Taking the pulp of fresh amla or amla juice with honey or ghee in morning and evening sharpens the intellect and invigorates the body.

(iv) Taking one piece of amla murabba with a cup of plain milk (without sugar) regularly for few days cures general weakness and strengthens weakened brain.

Eye Ailments

(i) Taking amla daily in the morning or 1 tsp. amla powder with water at night improves eye-sight.

(ii) Washing the eyes with amla water (soak amla in water at night and strain it) in the morning-keeps eyes fresh, sparkling and improves eye-sight.

(iii) Washing the eyes with ground amla and TO powder water (soak amla and TO powder in water overnight and strain it) in the morning cures burning sensation in the eyes.

(iv) Applying pulp of amla on the head and washing the hair after massage helps in curing burning sensation in the eyes and heaviness of the head.

(v) Taking amla powder with milk cures ailment of the eyes like sight loss or cataract.

(vi) Washing the eyes with water having triphala powder cures trachoma and other ailments of the eyes.

(vil) Eating 10 gms. of triphala powder with 1 tsp. of honey everyday keeps eyes very healthy strong and sparkling.

(viii) Taking 1 tsp. triphala powder (harar, bahod and amla) mixed with half teaspoon of pure ghee everyday in the morning improves eye-sight cures weakness of the eyes or darkness coming bofore eyes.

Heart and Mental Weakness

(i) Taking amla murabba everyday in the morning cures physical and mental debility.

(ii) Taking fresh juice of amla mixed with water (in between-taking of food) removes weakness of body, mind and heart.

(iii) Massaging the scalp with amla oil before going to bed-removes mental weakness.

(iv) Taking amla powder with cow's milk or mishri (same quantity) with water gives relief in heart ailments.

(v) Taking arnla murabba everyday strengthens mental faculties and sharpens memory.

(vi) Applying paste made up of dried amla powder with kumkum, neelkamal and gulabjal cures headache.

(vii) Applying paste of juice of 2 or 3 amla or its pulp mixed with little rose-water and 3 or 4 pieces of kesar in it on affected parts for 15 minutes relieves the pain of migraine.

Night-Discharge

(i) Taking 10 gm. fresh amla juice with 1 gm. powdered haldi and honey morning and evening regularly cures night discharge.

(ii) Taking amla water (soak dried amla powder in 1:3 proportion in water for 12 hours, strain the water and mix 1 gm. haldi powder) regularly helps in curing night discharge.

Urinary Problems

(i) Taking 1 gm. amla powder, kalajeerg and 2 gm. ground mishri with cold water cures the habit of urinating in the bed at night.

(ii) Taking milk after eating fresh amla juice or dried amla powder with gur cures strangury.

(iii) Applying paste of amla near the navel helps in curing urinary problems.

(Iv) Boil 20 gen. pulp of dried amla in 160 gm. water till 40 gms. is left. Then mix 20 gen. gur in it drinking this helps in urinary problems.

(v) Taking crushed amla pulp (after straining it) mixed with mishri cures blood in urine.

(vi) Taking 20 gen. fresh amla juice with 10 gen. honey and water twice a day cures urinating problems.

Acidity

Licking one teaspoon of dried amla powder with honey or ghee after dinner checks acidity.

Leucorrhoea

(i) Taking 3 gm. powdered amla with 6 gen. honey everyday foe onp month cures this.

(ii) Taking-powder of amla seed with honey or mishri regularly helps in curing ft.

(iii) Taking 20 gm. fresh amla juice mixed with honey regularly for a month checks leucorrhoea.

Blood Impurities

(i) Taking fresh amla juice or amla powder in tablet form checks impurities of blood.

(ii) Taking 5 gms. of powder (made from 20 gms. triphala, 20 gms. black pepper, 10 gms. pure sulphur, 5 gms. of neem leaves and mehandi leaves-ground In fine powder form) with a glass of water twice a day-cures all impurities in blood.

Diabetes

Taking fresh amla juice with honey checks diabetes.

Piles

(i) Soak 15 gms. amla and 15 gen. mehndi leaves in. 400 gen. water overnight strain it. Drinking this water checks piles.

(ii) Taking 5 gm. of triphala churna with a glass of whey-helps in curing piles.

(iii) Taking fresh amla jůice with 1 tsp. ghee, 1 tsp. honey and 100 gen of milk after lunch cures chronic piles.

Stone in Urinary Bladder

Taking Amla powder with radish helps in checking stone in bladder, breaking the stones and throwing ft out with urine.

Diarrhoea

(i) Taking fresh amla leaves with whey cures loose motions due to indigestion.

(ii) Taking juice of 5 fresh amlas with glucose or grape juice checks diarrhoea.

(iii) Rubbing the juice of amla on the gums of child helps in checking loose motions due to teething problem.

(iv) Swallowing dried amla powder and kaala namak (equal quantity) with water cures loose motions.

Dysentery

Taking 20 gms. of fresh amla juice with 5 gms. honey and 100 gms. of milk 3 or 4 times a day helps in curing dysentery.

Constipation

(i) Taking 1 tsp. dried amla powder with milk or water before sleep at night helps in discharging bowels easily.

(ii) Taking strained water of meshed fresh amlas soaked overnight in lukewarm water, helps in evacuating the bowels.

(iii) Taking 4 tsp. fresh amla juice and 3 tsp. honey mixed in a glass of water relieves constipation.

Worms

Taking about 20 gm. fresh amla juice daily kills worms.

Cough and Cold

(i) Taking two tsp. of fresh amla juice with honey twice a day helps in taking out the phlegm and controls cold.

(ii) Taking milk in which a little amla powder and ghee is boiled in the evening-helps in dry cough.

(iii) Licking amla powder with honey-regularly twice or thrice a day cures chronic dry cough.

Chronic Fever

Eating mung ki dal with dried amla powder cooked in it controls chronic fever.

Dryness in the Body

Taking tea boiled with pieces of ainla in it mixed with sugar and milk cures dryness of skin.

Itching

Applying amla churna in chameli oil (dry amlas in shade, powder and mix in chameli oil. The bottle should be kept in shade) on the part of the body where itching is there gives relief.

Baldness

Washing the head with amla juice mixed water after rubbing the scalp for 10-15 minutes with fresh amla juice-helps in growing of hair cuts. Applying fresh Amla juice on the wound caused by the cut-stops bleeding -and is an antiseptic.

High Blood Pressure

Taking juice of fresh amla or murabba amla everyday in the morning controls high blood pressure.

Anaemia

Taking 1 cup amla juice, 2 tsp. honey with little water regularly helps in curing anaemia.

Stammering

Taking one raw fresh amla everyday relieves stammering in children.

Nose Bleeding

(i) Taking amla ka murabba everyday helps in curing bleeding of nose.

(ii) Washing the hair with water in which dried amlas have been soaked overnight-gives relief.

(iii) Putting drop of fresh amla juice in the nostril or smelling the juice or applying the paste of amla on the forehead helps in checking the flow of blood.

THIRST DUE TO DEHYDRATION

Taking amla juice with grape juice or honey in the form of

sharbat quenches thirst and cures dehydration caused by diarrhoea, dysentery.

Hair Loss and Other Problems

(i) Soak dried amla, harer, baher and shikakal in an iron utensil overnight mesh them nicely. Washing regularly with this strengthens the hair, imparts glow and lustre, smoothness and blackness and also stops excessive hair fall.

(ii) Applying the paste of dried amla and mehandi leaves on the hair 10 or 15 minutes before washing make the hair black and strong.

(iii) Applying the paste of amla powder mixed in lemon juice on the hair 10 or 15 minutes before washing with amla water keeps the hair strong and shining.

(iv) Washing the hair with decoction of amla removes dryness of the scalp, checks dandruff and stops excessive fall and greying of hair.

(v) Massaging the head with amla oil imparts natural glow to hair, relieves mental tensions and induces sleep jaundice).

Digestive Problems

(i) Taking 10 gms. fresh amla juice with 10 gms. pomegranate juice, 20 gm. jaggery and 2 ground cloves (a) early in the morning before breakfast and (b) after food-cures constipation, wind-problems, other effects of indigestion.

(ii) Taking two tsp. of fresh amla juice mixed with two tsp. sugar or 2 tsp. dried amla powder mixed with same arnount of mishri with water cures this.

(iii) Taking amla juice morning and evening-cures chronic indigestion.

(iv) Eating raw amla on empty stomach everyday is very useful for the digestive system.

(v) Taking dried amla powder and little kaala namak with lukewarm water in summer and with honey in winter after meals cures all digestive problems.

Jaundice

(i) Soak 4 munakkas in juice of 4 fresh amla. After one hour grind the soaked munakkas and mix it with amla juice taking this twice a day gives relief in Jaundice.

(ii) Taking and licking little chuma (made by grinding 10 gms. each of amla, dry ginger, black pepper, 3 gm. of iron bhasm and little turmeric) with honey-cures Jaundice.

Gout

Taking fresh amla juice with old ghee-heated a little-regularly for few days relieves stiffness of joints and helps in curing gout.

Itching, burning-after measles chicken pox, small pox:

(i) Taking bath with water having fresh amla juice in it or having amlas boiled in it-relieves the itching and burning sensation after measles or chicken pox.

(ii) Apply the paste made of amla and til in equal quantity ground in cold milk added with 3 or 4 drops of rose water on spots and let it stay for sometime and then wash. This helps in removing the spots.

Boils in Mouth

Doing gargles with water having fresh arnla juice-twice or thrice a day givcs rclicf. After gargles apply fresh amla juice on the boils and let saliva ooze out.

Giddiness, Darkness Before Eyes

(i) Taking fresh amla juice with honey in the morning-cures this.

(ii) Taking harar, bahar and amla churna (triphala) in one tsp. mixed with ½ tsp. of pure ghee-in the morning helps in improvement of eye-sight and curing of giddiness, darkness etc.

(iii) Licking one tsp. of powdered amla with 1 tsp. of honey morning and evening-gives strength to the body and cures darkness before eyes.

Lices in Hair

Applying the paste of ground seeds of amla mixed with juice of lemon-on the roots of the hair, and washing after half an hour will clear the lices.

Obesity

Drinking a glass of amla water (in which Amlas have been soaked overnight) with 1 tsp. of honey early in the morning helps in slimming.

Menstrual Disorder

(i) Taking boiled pulp of amla with honey two times a day relieves one of very scanty and painful bleeding.

(ii) Taking amla juice mixed with ripe banana 3 or 4 times a day during periods checks profuse bleeding.

Insect Bite

(i) Applying the paste made of triphala powder mixed with cow's urine on the affected pan-relieves the poisonous effect of insects.

(ii) Drinking of amla juice is also very helpful.

Beauty Treatment

(i) Applying paste of amla mixed with turmeric and oil on the body makes the skinclear, soft and improm the comploxion..

(ii) Drinking amla juice (amlas to be soaked overnight crushed and then strained) mixed with honey in the moming makes the complexion full of natural glow and charm.

(iii) Applying the paste of soaked wet seeds of amla on the face eliminates pimples and g;ves natural beauty.

We find that amla is one of the important ingredients of *'triphala'* (i.e. harar, bahad and amla) out of which many ayurved drugs are made. It is really a rich storehouse of medicinal properties, helpful in eliminating and curing various physical and mental weakness and ailments. Apart from this use amla can also be used as food-item in different forms:

(i) Munching raw amla or one piece of amla Murabba followed by milk is an ideal breakfast for persons of all age groups.

(ii) Taking chutney or pickle of amla with meals is invigorating and digestive.

(iii) Taking chyavanaprash in the morning with milk is the best tonic for one and all.

(iv) Taking sharbat of amla especially in summer is refreshing and is a tonic.

Amla, undoubtedly, is capable of imparting glow and lustre and physical, mental strength and vigour to different parts of the body and also eliminating various diseases. It is an efficacious and extremely cheap 'Amrit Phala', which could be used by rich and poor alike for healthy long life.

10

Home Treatment by Papaya

In this chapter the mention of Papaya diet is often used. This means that Papaya should be more frequently used in our daily diet.

To maintain health the ripe fruit flesh is consumed and sometimes young Papaya sprouts incorporated in salads and vegetables.

Please note to avoid unnecessary repeating in the following text I have only mentioned, for example, compresses, oils, vinegar and so on. The methods of use and the production of the remedies are detailed in the chapter Home Made Papaya Medicine.

Abortion: The natives of tropical America and in the south sea islands used Papaya regularly to abort.

Acne: Fresh latex is used to treat affected areas. A mask using the fleshy side of the skin using a half ripe Papaya on the acne areas is also recommended. Papaya diet supports the treatment internally. Pickled grated papaya in vinegar, is used weekly as a mask. As a skin cleanser papaya vinegar is diluted 1:10. Stubborn areas are treated with undiluted papaya vinegar and Papaya oil.

Allergy to Papaya Pollen: Homeopathic papaya D6 (6x).

Allergies: Insufficient digestion may be the cause or trigger for some allergies and the papaya diet is recommended.

I have written several books and received many letters about home remedies people have used. When nothing else helps, the best remedy seems to be urine therapy. In some cases even homeopathic urine (your own - of course!) has been more successful than any other treatment. For more information about the wonders of urine therapy - I recommend that you read my book urine The holy water.

***Arterial hardening*:** Papaya diet, see also guava.

***Arthritis*:** Papaya diet; papaya tincture; kombucha papaya concentrate; papaya vinegar added to the bath water; guava-papaya concentrate; guava leaf tea; warm compresses with papaya vinegar; papaya oil.

***Ashma*:** Eat the ripe fruit flesh together with the seeds and skin in the morning on an empty stomach. In remote areas of Mexico the leaf is smoked to assist with asthma.

Asthma may be caused from your own home environment like earthrays, electromagnetic fields and others. The book *Pollution Sollution* by Harald W. Tietze, shows how to detect and avoid the cause of many illnesses.

***Bleeding, Stopping of*:** In India. latex is used to stop bleeding.

Bloating: Regular papaya diet; kombucha papaya concentrate: mature green papaya fruit.

***Blood Clots after Operation*:** Papaya diet; papaya vinegar added to the bath water.

***Blood Cleansing*:** Papaya diet; papaya flower essences: papaya skin extract; kombucha papaya concentrate; papaya vinegar added to the bath water.

***Blood Pressure—High*:** Papaya diet; papaya flower essences: papaya vinegar added to the bath water; guava tea: guava fruit. Hawthorn tea and fermented hawthorn tea have shown many good results.

***Blood Sugar too Low*:** See hypoglycaemia.

***Blood in Urine*:** A tea is made from the root by decoction and a cupful is taken three times daily.

***Bronchitis*:** Juice of the ripe fruit is cooked with honey or sugar, tea, made from the male flowers, is taken and sweetened with honey—one tablespoonful every hour is recommended.

***Burns*:** Latex is applied immediately to the burnt area. Not everyone always has fresh latex available, however, in my opinion the best, simplest, fastest and most effective method is to use fresh urine, I have also learned that another treatment is fresh aloe vera jelly and I now have aloe vera plants in areas such as the kitchen and workshop and if an accident happens the jelly is immediately available fresh from the leaf.

Cancer—Papaya as Cancer Medicine?

Only three years ago Papaya was known to me simply as a tropical fruit which, when added to lemon juice, had a positive effect on the digestion. Its medical qualities were only made aware to me through a woman who had written a letter to the German newspaper in Australia, "Die Woche". In this letter, the woman intended to communicate her success with papaya as a possibility to cancer sufferers. Mrs H. had already lost any hope for being healed until she was made aware of Papaya leaves and their possible positive effect. In her letter she mentions that the healing of her cancer was because of the papaya leaves.

A more detailed report is found in the "*Weekend Bulletin*" (Gold Coast. Australia) which deals with the healing of bladder cancer of Mrs K, a 74 year old woman. Mrs K had an operation however, the cancer could not be completely removed which is why she was supposed to have further treatment in Brisbane. Over a period of three months she used papaya leaves. and as she ran out of leaves, she used the skin of the fruit which she boiled. When she went back to the doctor for a further check-up after that period. the diagnosis was that the cancer had been healed. A check-up four months later confirmed the original result. Reports confirm that Mrs. K is feeling 100% and she sees her result as proof that papaya has the ability to heal cancer.

There are many reports that cancer sufferers have been healed by drinking papaya leaf concentrate. A kombucha-fermented papaya leaf extract is available in health shops. Kombucha concentrate is now manufactured in Australia. During further research on this subject, I was able to find several health practitioners who for some time had already used papaya in the fight against cancer. Unfortunately none of them were able to give me any details. fearing legal implications.

In the Gold Coast Bulletin, several reports were issued, "Pawpaw's medicilnal qualities" and "Pawpaw cancer plea bears fruit". Please note that in Australia Papaya is called Pawpaw. The first indications regarding the healing capabilities of papaya were made in 1978. With many people now using this method in the battle against cancer the leaves are now becoming rare.

The most common recipe for papaya leaf juice

Use seven medium size papaya leaves not very old ones, and not too young.

The leaves should be washed thoroughly and partly dried. Cut them up like cabbage and put them in a saucepan together with 2 litres of water.

Bring the water and leaves to the boil and simmer (without a lid) until the water is reduced by half.

Strain the liquid and bottle in glass containers.

a. The concentrate will keep in the refrigerator for three to four days. If it becomes cloudy it should be discarded.

b. For Kombucha brewing the concentrate is mixed together with green tea or other medicinal teas to one's needs.

Kombucha fermentation conserves the properties of the papaya leaves in a natural way.

The recommended dosage in the original recipe is 50 ml three times a day. The concentrate can also be added to other juices.

If papaya concentrate is fermented together with other teas the dosage is calculated on the proportion. For example if 1 litre of papaya concentrate and 1 litre of green tea is fermented together the calculated dosage is 100 ml three times a day.

Some people use the semi-mature (mature green) papaya fruit (with seeds and skin), which is said to have the same healing effect as the papaya leaves. The papaya can be processed in a kitchen blender and can be mixed with other fruits.

***Candida*:** Papaya diet; papaya vinegar.

***Catarrh of the Stomach*:** A tea is prepared from the root and three cups a day are taken.

***Children Growing and Low on Energy*:** Ripe fruit is incorporated into the papaya diet: papaya vinegar is added to the bath water.

***Colic*:** Papaya diet used as a preventative if colic is frequent: latex diluted is used for colic: papaya flower essence, papaya skin extract. compresses with papaya and massages with papaya oil. **Caution** overdoses of unripe fruit with seeds and skin can cause colic as I personally have experienced.

***Constipation*:** Papaya is very effective even in cases of chronic constipation and is safe to take when incorporated into the diet. Most other treatments, chemical or natural, have negative side effects. Other treatments with papaya are warm compresses: massages with papaya oil; Kombucha papaya concentrate.

***Corns*:** Latex is applied.

***Cough Chronic*:** A juice of the ripe fruit is cooked with honey or sugar; papaya tincture; inhalations of Papaya vinegar: massages with papaya oil, Kombucha Papaya Concentrate.

***Croup*:** Diluted latex: papaya diet: papaya vinegar added to the bath water: massages with papaya oil.

***Dairy Food Intolerance*:** Papaya diet: Papaya Kombucha Concentrate: skin extract.

***Dandruff*:** Hair is washed with diluted latex skin extract for the first wash diluted papaya vinegar mixed with lemon juice is used and left for 20 minutes. The hair is rinsed with diluted papaya vinegar. A papaya hair shampoo is manufactured by Kneipp Cure in Australia.

***Diabetes*:** The ripe fruit together with the seeds and skin is taken: Papaya vinegar added to the bath water: Guava-Papaya Concentrat; Guava leaf tea.

Diarrhoea: Papaya diet. In South America 20 grams of the green fruit or young shoots are cooked in half a litre of water. One cup of this tea is taken three times daily with main meals, papaya,

Guava Leaf Concentrate.

Digestive Problems: Papaya diet: skin extract: warm compresses with papaya vinegar: Kombucha papaya concentrate.

***Discs Herniated Lumbar Intervertebral*:** In the United States of America, the F.D.A. have approved direct injections of a Papaya product for patients who have had no improvement of their condition through other common treatments.

***Diverticulosis*:** Long term Papaya diet is said to be of benefit.

Caution: The seeds should not be taken with Diverticulosis.

***Dysentery*:** 15 - 20 grams of green fruit is cooked in half a litre of water—three cups are taken daily with main meals; cold compresses with papaya vinegar. In Mexico and Jamaica the ripe food with seeds and skin is taken. In other areas only the ripe fruit flesh is taken but it is stressed thaf it has to be taken regularly and in large quantities.

***Elephantitis, Elephantoid Growths*:** Poulticed leaves are used for treatment as well as the fresh latex.

***Emmenagogue*:** Semi-mature fruit flesh is taken.

***Energy—Low*:** Low energy can be caused by poor digestion, papaya diet supporting digestion is of benefit; skin extract; papaya vinegar added to the bath water; foot bath with Papaya vinegar, papaya Kombucha concentrate.

***Epilepsy*:** papaya diet. It is reported that attacks are less frequent.

guava-papaya concentrat; Guava leaf tea; massages with guava oil or tincture.

***Fat—body*:** The green Papaya fruit is regularly incorporated in the Papaya diet; Papaya vinegar is added to the bath water; Kombucha Papaya Concentrate.

***Feet—Inflammation of*:** In China, dried pulp of the green fruit is used.

***Fever*:** Papaya diet: to reduce high fever—compresses with Papaya vinegar on the lower legs, changed every 30 minutes are very effective. If no papaya vinegar is available, common vinegar may be used.

Flu: papaya diet; papaya tea; Papaya vinegar added to the bath. water; compresses with Papaya vinegar; skin extract, Papaya kombucha concentrate.

Fungal Growths: The affected areas are treated with latex or strong papaya leaf tea. Compresses or washings with papaya vinegar are also used.

Gall Stones: See Gravel.

Gastritis: Depending on the degree of the problem. ripe fruit or green fruit is taken. The green fruit is stronger. papaya tincture: papaya skin extract; Papaya flower essence.

Gout: Papaya diet: Kombucha papaya concentrate: skin extract: compresses with papaya vinegar; papaya vinegar added to the bath water; papaya oil.

Gravel: In Java, it is said that papaya diet prevents gravel and that small kidney and gall stones are dissolved. Papaya kombucha concentrate.

Haematuria: See Blood in urine.

Haemorrhoids: In some countries the roots are bashed and barked and placed on the haemorrhoids. In other countries fresh latex is used.A cotton ball is soaked in papaya oil and is placed on the haemorrhoids.

A friend of mine, had problems with his haemorrhoids as the high pressure of the water caused him unbearable pain whilst diving in deep water. A piece of cotton soaked in the oil solved the problem and enabled him to continue with his occupation without pain.

Hay Fever: Papaya diet is reported to be beneficial in many cases of hay fever; inhaling of papaya vinegar.According to some specialists, the best treatment for hay fever if nothing else has helped is urine therapy. In some cases homeopathic urine was even more successful than anything else tried before.

Heart Nervous: The seeds are taken or incorporated in cooking. For faster relief seeds are ground and taken together with honey. If there are no seeds available - young shoots and leaves may be used as well as skin extract: papaya tea; papaya vinegar added to the bath water. The heart area is massaged with papaya oil.

***Heart—Weak*:** Papaya diet; papaya flower essences; papaya tea: skin extract papaya vinegar added to the bath water.

***Heartburn*:** Ripe fruit is eaten for prevention or at the time of heartburn - papaya tea is drunk; kombucha papaya concentrate: mature green papaya fruit. .

***Hypertension*:** Papaya diet; the seeds are ground, mixed with honey and taken several times a day.

***Hypoglycaemia*:** Papaya diet; papaya vinegar is added to the, bath water; papaya tea is taken several times a day.

***Immune System Improvement*:** Papaya diet; papaya essence; skin extract; papaya vinegar added to the bath water: massages with Papaya oil, papaya kombucha concentrate.

***Indigestion*:** Papaya diet; papaya tincture; kombucha papaya concentrate; skin extract.

***Infections*:** External infections and ulcers are treated with latex. Very thin slices of the green fruit or mashed leaves are used as well. For internal treatments young leaves are cooked like a vegetable andl the water is taken as a tea: Kombucha Papaya Concentrate; Papaya vinegar added to the bath water, compresses with Papaya vinegar, skin extract: papaya powder taken as a tea.

***Insect bites*:** Latex or papaya vinegar is rubbed on the insect bite.

***Intestinal Infection*:** Papaya diet: papaya flower extract; Kombucha Papaya Concentrate: compresses with Papaya vinegar; skin extract.

***Intestinal Parasites*:** See Worms.

***Itch*:** The affected areas are treated with latex or with the fleshy side of the skin. Compresses with papaya vinegar papaya oil; papaya vinegar added to the bath water.

***Jaundice*:** Small root pieces are cooked for 20 minutes in the water and three times a day one cupful is drunk before meals.The natives in tropical south sea islands eat the flowers.

***Jelly Fish Poisoning*:** Fresh latex or papaya vinegar is rubbed immediately onto the affected area.

***Kidney Stones*:** See Gravel.

***Laryngitis*:** In tropical countries a tea is made from male flowers and sweetened with honey—one tablespoonful every hour is recommended. Fresh juice made from the ripe papaya (without seed) is taken and sweetened with honey. If the treatment doesn't bring fast enough relief the juice of a half ripe or green papaya is taken with honey. Compresses with papaya vinegar; gargling with papaya vinegar; external massages to the throat with papaya oil.

***Labour, Trigger of*:** In Asia, latex is smeared on the mouth of uterus to trigger labour.

***Liver Enlargement*:** papaya diet, papaya kombucha concentrate.

***Longevity*:** The natives of tropical countries see papaya as a longevity fruit. Considering the illnesses of our modern civilisations the natives might be right.

***Lymphatic Congestion*:** Papaya vinegar is added to the bath water compresses with papaya vinegar; massages with papaya oil. Papaya Kombucha Concentrate.

Some doctors came to the conclusion that lymphatic congestion is caused by mucoprotein built up in the interstitial spaces which have developed over a long period of time. Green Papaya cooked as a vegetable reduces the build up in the intestines and all this stage has had positive results with this problem.

***Menstrual Irregularities*:** Women who have problems getting their menstruation regularly often find relief eating the green papaya as a vegetable. The seeds and the skin of the papaya is in this case not consumed. Papaya flower essence; skin extract and papaya vinegar is added to the bath water; massages of the lower abdomen with the papaya oil.

In Peru and in some south sea islands the green fruit is used for irregular menstruation, or early pregnancy which is aborted by taking the fruit with the skin and the seed.

***Milk—Stimulation of, After Child Birth*:** The ripe fruit is incorporated into the papaya diet. In South America women massage their breasts with thin slices of green papaya fruit for stimulation of the milk glands. Papaya diet gives energy and is a tonic for breast feeding mothers and growing children. Stinging nettle tea has shown very good results in stimulating milk flow as well.

***Mouth Hygiene*:** Papaya tea after meals.

***Mucus*:** Papaya diet; skin extract; papaya vinegar; Kombucha papaya concentrate papaya leaf, mature green papaya fruit.

***Obesity*:** Papaya diet; skin extract: Kombucha Papaya Concentrate: papaya vinegar added to the bath water; massages with Papaya oil.

***Oliguria*:** Papaya juice mixed with lemon juice is taken. In South America, 4 young leaves are cooked in 1litre of water one cupful is taken three times a day with meals.

***Pain*:** Poulticed leaves or the skin, preferably warmed up, are applied to the painful areas; massages with Papaya vinegar or papaya oil, papaya-guava leaf concentrate; guava tea.

***Pancreas Problems*:** Specialist Dr Alfred Vogel recommends Papaya products for the support of the pancreas together with the herb Lady's Bedstraw (gallium verum): Guava tea; Guava-Papaya Concentrat.

***Parasites—Internal*:** Scc worms.

***Piles*:** See Haemorrhoids

***Psoriasis*:** Papaya diet: latex; compresses with papaya vinegar: Papaya Kombucha Concentrate; papaya vinegar added to the bath water; massaging with papaya oil.

The fruit (with the skin) is grated and placed into a jar with lemon juice, salt water (15% - 150 grams per litre of water) is then filled into the jar until the pieces are covered. The jar is stored in a cool spot. It helps in curing psorisis.

***Rheumatism*:** In Japan, eating the ripe fruit for rheumatism is recommended; warm compresses with papaya vinegar.

***Ringworms*:** See worms.

Roundworms: See Worms.

Scorpion Stings: Fresh latex is used immediately on the sting.

Sex Drive: Large amounts of Papaya consumed can, have a calming effect on the sex drive. Normal sensible consumption on the other hand has a slight positive effect especially with nervous people. People with digestive problems may find that papaya increases the sex drive. Skin extract; flower essences.

Skin - brown spots: The spots are treated daily with fresh latex; papaya vinegar; papaya oil.

Skin cancer: There are quite a number of quite successful treatments with Papaya of skin cancer.

In the first instance latex is used on the cancerous areas. Natives in tropical countries use poulticed leaves on the skin cancer which sticks to the skin with the gluey latex. This treatment is applied several times daily.

Slimming : Papaya diet, papaya Kombucha Concentrate.

Spleen enlargement: Regular consumption of ripe fruit flesh is recommended.

In India the ripe fruit flesh is used without seeds and skin. It is cut into cubes and stored in vinegar, for a week. For treatment approximately 20 grams are consumed twice daily. If the illness was caused by malaria then the fresh fruit flesh is used and taken together with cumin and pepper.

Swellings: Latex is applied to the swelling. The skin of unripe fruit with the fleshy side to the swelling is also used. Compresses with papaya vinegar are also applied.

Syphilis: In Africa, tea from the root is made by infusion which is then taken regularly over a long period of time.

Throat disorders: Tea is made from the male flowers and sweetened with honey to taste. One tablespoon is taken hourly.

Fresh juice made from the ripe papaya, using the skin but not the seeds, is sweetened to taste with honey and taken. Should this not bring fast relief the juice of a half mature or green papaya, sweetened with honey as well, is taken. Compresses with papaya vinegar; gargling with papaya vinegar; Papaya oil is massaged on the throat externally.

Tonsils—enlarged: Gargling with diluted latex. Papaya tea or Papaya vinegar. Natives eat the green fruit.

Tooth hygiene: Papaya tea made from the leaves drunk after meals.

Toothaches: In Peru, the inner bark of the tree is placed in the mouth on the painful area; guava tea leaf.

Tuberculosis: Papaya diet.

Tumour of the uterus: Sinapisms prepared from the root.

Tumour: Papaya diet preferably of unripe fruit. young shoots and leaves, papaya Kombucha concentrate, guava leaf tea.

Ulcer—peptic and stomach: Papaya diet; papaya flower essence: skin extract; homeopathic papaya D3 (3x).

Caution: High dosages of green papaya as it is sometimes taken by people with cancer may have negative side-effects.

Ulcers—external: The skin is applied with the pulp side down on the ulcer. Green papaya is more effective than ripened papaya.

Under nourishment: The ripe fruit with the seeds and skin is eaten with honey added to taste.

Urine concretions: Papaya vinegar; Kombucha papaya concentrate; papaya tea.

Urine—acidity reducing of: Papaya diet.

Warts: Treated several times a day with fresh latex. The warts will disappear over several days. Another good remedy for getting rid of warts is by using the skin of a banana. Place the soft inside of the skin on the warts and renew it several times a day and they will disappear after a few days. This still works even if the banana skin is only applied overnight after work. A lady had a very big wart on the index finger and was embarrassed to shake hands. however, with the banana skins only applied overnight she was able to get rid of the wart within a few days. That was six months ago and to date the wart has not returned.

Worms—all & other intestinal parasites of the intestines: The worm plague in the intestines is widely underestimated. There are many remedies on the market but papaya seems to be the best remedy for eliminating all intestinal parasites at one time without negative side-effects. Papaya and minerals are mentioned in the contents and is probably enough to stay worm free. "Stubborn worms" need a more concentrated treatment. The most common method is to mix 20 ground papaya seeds with the same weight of honey in a glass of warm water which is then taken on an empty stomach for four days in a row. The seeds contain caricin to expel the worms.

In tropical countries fresh leaves are eaten to alleviate worms in the intestines. The alkaloid carpain in the leaves kills some worms and others are expelled.

In India, they have a lot of problems with intestinal parasites and I have found the following a very good treatment. One tablespoon latex, one tablespoon honey and four tablespoons hot water are mixed together and taken on an empty stomach. After taking this mixture meals may be taken. Two hours later a mixture of 50 ml castor oil and 300 ml warm milk are taken. This treatment is taken for three days in a row. Children between 6 and 12 years of age take only half the dosage and for children under 3 or 4 years a teaspoonl of the mixture is given.

Wounds—foul: Dressing with fresh poulticed leaves after cleaning with latex.

11

Home Treatment by Turmeric

Turmeric is stringent and sour in taste. It is a time-tested beauty aid and a nourishing herb which not only gives natural gloss, royal glow and lustre but also imparts vigour and youthful vitality to the entire body. Turmeric is thus a great tonic in general, aromatic, diuretic, expectorant, blood-purifier, skin tonic, carminative, pain reliever, germicidal, anti-flatulent, producer and enhancer of red blood corpuscles, anti-phlegmatic, antibilleous, protector of eyes, anti-inflammatory and imparts coolness to the system.

Bruises, Sprain and Wounds

(i) Applying pasts of turmeric powder with lime or water on the effected part eliminates swelling and pain in bruises.

(ii) Taking 1 tsp. turmeric powder with hot milk is also useful.

(iii) Filling the wound or cut, (from which blood is coming out) with Turmeric powder will stop bleeding and curing of the wound/cut.

(iv) Applying poultice made of gram flour, turmeric powder mixed with mustard or til oil-on the sprained portion enhances blood circulation and gives relief.

(v) Tying a bandage of turmeric (prepared with 4 tsp. flour, 2 tsp. turmeric powder, 1 tsp. pure ghee, ½ tsp. sendha namak with water) on the bruised portion gives relief.

(vi) Giving fomentation with cloth soaked in hot water (500 gm. water boiled with 1 tsp. sendha namak and 1 tsp. turmeric powder) on the bruised part eliminates pain and swelling.

(vii) Giving fomentation with Potli (having one ground onion mixed with 1 tsp. turmeric powder) heated with Til oil on the bruised portion gives relief.

(viii) Applying turmeric powder heated in ghee or oil on the wound and tying it with a bandage helps in quick healing of the wound.

(ix) Dusting turmeric powder on wounds also helps.

Skin Problems

(i) Ringworm white spots applying paste of turmeric rubbed on stone with water on the effected portion is useful.

(ii) Applying paste of Turmeric and til oil on the body prevents skin eruptions.

(iii) Applying turmeric powder or paste on the body before bath is a preventive against skin problems and also a depilatory (clears the growth of hair on body).

(iv) Taking 1 tsp. turmeric powder with 1 tsp. mishri or honey twice a day cures urticaria.

Taking halwa (made from 2 tsp. flour, 1 tsp. ghee, tsp. turmeric, 2 tsp sugar, 1 cup water) in the morning cures Utricaria.

(v) Tiking roasted turmeric with gur cures itching.

(vi) Sucking tablet of ground haldi with honey for 10- 15 days cures Eczema.

(vii) Placing cotton dipped in turmeric oil over pustules gives relief.

(viii) Applying turmeric rubbed on stone with water eliminates freckles and spots.

Massaging the face with Ubtan (mix ground Turmeric with milk of banyan or pipal & soak it overnight) 1 hour before bath eliminates freckles on the face and imparts natural glow.

Cough & Cold, Asthma

(i) Taking haldi powder and little salt with hot water or sucking a small piece of turmeric or licking 1 tsp. turmeric powder with ¼ tsp. honey gives relief in 4 cough and eliminates congestion of bronchi.

(ii) Taking ¼ tsp. turmeric with hot milk is helpful in checking running nose.

(iii) Inhaling the smoke of burnt turmeric throws out the trapped phlegm.

(iv) Taking ¼ tsp. powder of turmeric (roasted in hot sand and then ground) with hot water relieves breathing problem (Asthma).

(v) Taking turmeric boiled in milk and sweetened with jaggery is very useful in cold and Asthma.

(vi) Sucking a piece of turmeric (like lemon drops) or keeping it in mouth at night cures chronic cold.

(vii) Licking tablets (made by mixing turmeric powder, barley powder and bansa-ash in equal proportion and honey and. making small tablets) 4-5 times in a day eliminates trapped phlegm in the body.

(viii) Massaging the throat & chest with little turmeric powder, ground black pepper mixed with ghee cures irritation In bronchial chords.

(ix) Giving a pinch of turmeric powder with milk to children gives quick relief.

(x) Inhaling smoke of cow dung cake with turmeric sprinkled on it releases the trapped phlegm.

(xi) Taking ¼ tsp. of turmeric powder with 3-4 gulps of warm water-acts as a preventive against attack of Asthma.

Whooping cough

(i) Taking 1 tsp. ground roasted turmeric powder with two spoons of honey 3 or 4 times a day gives relief in cough.

(ii) Taking pan with little turmeric piece in it is also useful.

Indigestion & Stomach Problems

(i) Taking turmeric powder and salt in equal quantity with warm water gives instant relief in acidity.

(ii) Taking 1 tsp. churna (grind turmeric 4 gm., sonth 4 gm., black pepper 2 gm. and ilayachi 2 gm.) after meals is digestive, eliminates wind and stomach ailments.

(iii) Taking curd or whey with turmeric powder after lunch cures digestive problems.

Sore-Throat

Licking turmeric powder mixed with honey 2-3 times a day cures soreness.

Tonsilitis

Fomentation with paste made of 10 gm. turmeric powder roasted in mustard oil and then tied around the neck gives relief in tonsils.

Blisters in Mouth

Gargling with I glass water in which little turmeric powder is boiled, twice a day, cures it.

Urinary Troubles

Taking paste of ground or juice of raw turmeric and honey with goat's milk (if available) twice a day, cures all urinary problems.

Smallpox

(i) Taking! tsp. powder of turmeric and imli (tamarind) for 4-5 days acts as a preventive against small-pox.

(ii) Applying a thin layer of the ubtan (turmeric powder, foam of fresh milk and wheat flour mixed with mustard oil or fresh cream) on the affected part twice a day-flattens the deep spots of small-pox and makes the skin soft.

Worms

Licking the paste (made of ¼ tsp. turmeric powder and ½ tsp. vayavidang choorna with 1 tsp. of honey-for 7-8 days kills worms and throws them out.

Pregnancy and Postnatal Care

(i) Taking 5-10 gms. of turmeric powder with water during menses is an antipregnancy dose for ladies.

(ii) Taking 1 tsp. with hot milk in latter part of the 9th month of pregnancy helps in easy delivery.

(iii) Taking 1 tsp. roasted turmeric powder with gur after delivery eliminates weakness and cures uterus swelling.

Pain in Breasts

Applying paste of turmeric rubbed on stone on the affected part eliminates pain.

Gout

Taking laddu of turmeric (mix ½ kg. roasted ground turmeric, one fincly grated dried coconut 1 kg. jaggery, 200 gm. cashew nuts or ground nuts and make laddu) daily in the morning with tulsi or lemon tea makes the joints supple and gives relief in pain and swelling.

Pain in Ribs

(i) Applying paste of turmeric powder mixed in hot water on the aching ribs gives relief or

(ii) Massaging the ribs with turmeric oil or

(iii) Massaging the ribs with paste of turmeric powder in milk of the aak plant gives quick relief.

Jaundice & Liver Problems

Taking 4-5 gms. of turmeric powder mixed in a glass of whey twice a day activates the liver.

Diabetes

Taking 4-5 gms. ground turmeric with water or honey twice a day is helpful in curing diabetes.

Leucorrhoea

(i) Taking turmeric powder with sugar twice a day for sometime checks this.

(ii) Washing the private parts with turmeric water (10 gm. turmeric boiled in 100 gm. water) is also useful. Alongwith it taking one batasha with 8-10 drops of milk of banyan tree before sunrise for 7 days helps in early cure.

Debility in Males

Taking about 7-8 gms. of raw ground turmeric and equal amount of honey with aoat's milk referabi I cures debilltv in males.

Dental Problems

(i) Rinsing the mouth with turmeric water (boil 5 gms. turmeric powder, 2 clove and 2 dried leaves of guava in 200 gms. water) gives instant relief.

(ii) Applying and rubbing the teeth with paste of turmeric powder, salt and mustard oil strengthens the gums.

(iii) Massaging the aching teeth with roasted ground turmeric 41 iminates pain and swelling.

(iv) Keeping piece of roasted turmeric near the aching tooth and letting the saliva ooze out also helps.

(v) Filling the cavity in teeth-with roasted ground turmeric powder gives relief from pain.

(vi) Applying the powder of burnt turmeric piece and ajwain on teeth and cleaning them makes the gums and teeth strong.

Ear Troubles

Putting one or two drops of turmeric' (by roasting 2 pieces of turmeric in mustard oil) in the ear, cleaning it with an ear bud cures ear problems.

Eye Troubles

(i) Cloth dipped in the solution of turmeric powder and,water is employed as an eye-shade.

(ii) Dropping turmeric water (1 tsp. turmeric powder boiled in 500 gms. water till 125 gm. water is left. Cool and strain it through a fine cloth) in the eyes twice a day and putting the cotton soaked in water on the eyelids relieves pain, redness, irritation and itching in the eyes.

(iii) Applying, bit heated paste of piece of turmeric rubbed on stone on eyelids also eliminates pain, swelling and eye troubles.

(iv) A decoction of turmeric powder with water as a cooling lotion on the eyes is useful in conjunctivities.

Poison of Insect bite

Applying the mixture of turmeric powder and lime over the affected part nullifies the toxic effect.

Coryza

Inhalations of fumes of burning turmeric passed into the nostrils relieves coryza.

12

Home Treatment by Basil

Basil is the most sacred plant in Indian culture. This is loved by God's and a boon for human beings. One must cultivate a basil plant in his/her house to utilise its benefits.

Cataract

Extract the juice of Basil and add a little of honey to it. Apply this over the eye every morning and evening. If the cataract be of raw type, it shall be cut away and if it be of ripe type, it shall be ripened soon to enable the doctor to remove it by operation.

Cold and Cough

The chronic patient of this problem have their hair going untimely white. To stop the process and cure it, take 300 gms. of Basil leaves dried in shade, 50 gms. of dalchin, 100 gms. tejpat, 200 gms. sonff (aniseeds), 200 gms. of small cardamom, agiya 300 gms; Banfshaw 25 gms; red sandal 200 gms. and brahmi herb 200 gms grind all these ingredients and strain them through a cloth. Now take 10 gms. of this powder, boil it in 500 gms. water and when just a cup of this water remains, add sugar and milk and drink it twice a day like you have tea. All these problems will vanish in a couple of days.

Dirty Water purifying agent

Sometimes people don't like water of a new place. Just put a couple of Basil leaves and then you'd face no problems. If you put just two leaves of Basil in a pitcher of water for an hour or so, and then remove them, the water shall be purified immediately.

Ear Pain

Take about 10 leaves of Makoy and the leaves of Basil. Extract their juice together and put it in the affected ear when it is slightly lukewarm (heat it a little in the sn). Alternatively add half a tablet of camphor in Basil juice and put this juice in the ear for instant relief.

Eye Troubles

Put a drop of Basil juice mixed with even quantity of honey for all sort of eye troubles, especially pain and burning. This solution can also be preserved in a bottle. If there be the problem of trachoma, grind ten leaves of Basil together with a clove. Put it into your eyes every four hours. If there be swelling in the eyes, add a little of Basil-juice with alum and apply in your eyes for instant relief.

Epilepsy

Rub Basil juice over your body every day after taking your bath. Keep the blossoms of Basil inside the fold of your hanky every tiem. At the time of attack, smell the blossom deeply. Should the attack make one unconscious, grind 11 leaves of Basil, add a little salt to it and put a few drops of this juice in the patient's nostrils. He would immediately regain his consciousness.

Flatulence

Take about 10 gms. of Basil juice, 10 gms; of dry ginger and 20 gms. of jaggery. Mix all of them together to form small tablets. Take this tablet thrice a day with water to set right your digestive process. But during the period you have this trouble, better keep fast or take only easily digestible food.

Fistula

Have three or four Basil leaves every morning with water. Alternatively take the root of Basil plant and the fruit of Neem tree (Nimboli) and grind them togther. Take 2 gms. of this combination every morning with whey for quick relief.

Flu

Take about 10 gms. of Basil-leaves and 250 gms. of water. Boil them together till water is halved. Now add in the remaining water rock salt, according to taste. No sooner did you start to sweat that the effect of flu shall be removed with the sweat and you shall be alright. Alternatively drink karha of Basil leaves, black pepper and batasha for still quicker relief.

Hoarse Voice

Just extract the juice of 10 Basil leaves, add a little of honey and lick it. Just a small spoonful quantity of this solution will soothen your throat nerves and your voice will be again sweet.

Hair Trouble

Put about 21 leaves of Basil and 10 gms. of anwala churna in a big bowl. Add a little of water to make a paste of them. Apply it evenly on your head and allow it to dry. Then wash it with cold water. This will prevent hair loss and clear dandruff also.

Heart Troubles

Basil is very effective to cure all sort of heart troubles. Since it controls blood presure and keeps blood clean, its regualr consumption prevents heart attacks. For especial tonic for heart, prepare the medicine in the following way. Take about 1 gm. dried powder of Arjun tree and mix even amount of honey. Now either churn or mix them till the solution is fully homogeous. Take about 1 gm. of this paste, add a little more of honey and lick it at least thrice a day, preferably early in the morning as the first thing, an hour after lunch and as the last thing before you are retiring for the day.

Hysteria

If the hysteric effect be due to excess of phlegm in the body, make the patient smell Basil leaves and drink 5 Basil leaves juice. If it is caused by the excessive heat going to the head, grind five Basil leaves and five black pepper by mixing them in water and make the patient drink this water every morning and evening for a week's time. Hysteria will be cured.

Indigestion

Take the seeds of Basil and peepal in equal quantity and grind them to fine powder form. Now add 3 gms. of this powder with a spoonful of honey and lick it twice a day to clear indigestion. Drinking the tea of Basil leaves also brings quick relief. The filthy substance will get out of the body with sweat and urine. Alternatively add 1gm. of rock salt in 10 gms. of Basil leaves' paste and swallow it down with water.

Insomnia

The easiest and best treatment of this problem is to pluck 51 leaves of Basil. Give to patient just one leave for chewing it and spread rest of the leaves evenly below his pillow and the corners of bed below the bed sheet. As the smell of Basil leaves strikes his nostril, the pereson will feel sleepy and soon he will fall into sleep.

Icathing

Extract juice of Basil and massage on the parts of the body itching. If the trouble be chronic, take about 2 parts of Basil juice and one part of til oil. Allow them to parboil on slow fire. Then cool it and put it in a bottle. This is a most effective oil for all sorts of itching problems.

Jaundice

Add 10 gms. Basil-leaves' juice in about 50 gms. of radish juice. Add a little of jaggery to the combination to sweeten it. Have this solution twice or thrice daily for about a month for getting total relief from this problem.

Alternatively take 3 gms. of Basil-leaves' juice and 3 gms. of the root of Punarnava. Mix them both in 50 gms. of water and drink it for about 15 days. This is a very effective dose to cure Jaundice.

Kidney Troubles

For any type of kidney trouble, Basil-juice provides a very effective cure. Just soak 5 to 7 gms. of Basil seeds overnight in water. In the morning grind them with sugar and drink the combination. Soon the congestion or infection in kidney will be thrown out by means of copious discharge of urine.

Leprosy

Living in an atmosphere abounding with Basil plant is the best treatment. For white patches chew 5 leaves of Basil every morning, evening and afternoon. Licking the combination of Basil leaves' juice with honey will cure the trouble quickly.

Leucoderma

(i) Add a few drops of lime-juice in Basil-leaves' juice; (ii) grind 10 gms. Basil-leaves with a clove of garlic and apply the paste on the affected portion every day, 10 days for total relief.

Lethargy

The tea made of basil-leaves provides instant energy and makes one quite energetic. This is not a cumbersome preposition because as you prepare tea, so you prepare this Basil tea and instead of putting tea-leaves, put Basil leaves. The regular intake of this tea shall not only provide energy but will also keep you away from all the diseases borne out of the vitiation of kaph (phlegm) in the body.

Migraine

Get a small bunch of Basil blossom; dry it in the shade and grind it to powder form. Just take 2 gms. of it, mix 1/2 a spoonful of honey to it and make the person lick it. God willing, you may never require second dose, for it is a very efficacious treatment. In case you feel like, have another dose by the evening for a total cure.

Mouth Boils

Take just a leaf of Chameli plant, and four leaves of Basil. Chew them properly for a few minutes and suck in the juice. In about a day the trouble will vanish.

Malaria

Take about 10 gms. of Basil leaves' juice and add to it 1 gm. of ground black pepper. Administer this dose five or six days after every two hours. Alternatively make small tablets of this combination and feed the patient on Basil tea additionally. In a couple of days the fever will vanish alongwith the malarial infection.

Night Blindness

Put two drops of Basil leaves every morning and evening and drink the juice also at three times a day. Continue the treatment for about a month for total cure.

Black pepper is also very effective to cure this trouble. Put some black peppers' grain in a wet cloth to allow them to bloat up. Now remove their rinds and grind them in Basil juice. Line this paste in your eyes every morning and evening for total cure.

Nose-bleeding

The easiest and most effective cure of this trouble is to keep the Basil blossom near you and smell it as and when you like. For those who are chronic patient of this trouble, this simple treatment is very effective and cures the trouble almost totally. Drinking Basil juice mixed with honey will also help and provide extra strength to the body.

Paralysis

Boil a few leaves of Basil in a tumblerful of water. When cool, strain and put this water in a bottle. Massage this water on the affected limbs. Continue this treatment for at least two weeks. This treatment, coupled with regular intake of the Basil leaves will produce the desired results.

Pneumonia

Get the pure Basil oil from a recognised Ayurvedic medicine shop. Put this oil on the chest of the afflicted person. Together with this treatment, extract the juice of 5 Basil leaves, mix with it a few ground grains of black pepper at 6 hourly interval. This combined treatment will produce enough heat in the body to make the person sweat. With sweat all the effect of cold inside the body shall vanish and the patient will be cured.

Chicken pox

If the person be already afflicted with this problem, then giving Basil leaves' juice mixed with Ajwain (Bishop's seeds) will provide relief. But to prevent this menace afflicting you or your family members, prepare anti small pox tablets in the following way and administer one tablet daily with water.

Take 5 gms. Basil leaves, 2.5 gms. javitri,1/2 gm. real pearl ash, 20 grains black pepper, 1/2 gm. saffron and 1/4 gm. cloves. Add Ganga water to make these tablets.

Spleen Enlargement

Take 5 gms. Basil leaves dried under shade, 5 gms. Indra Jau and grind both of them to powder form. Add a little of salt and take the combination with a glass of cold water. Continue this treatment every morning and evening for 10 to 15 days. The effect of Basil leaves will bring spleen to size and cure the trouble.

Sluggish Liver

Take 5 Basil-leaves, 2 gms. roasted powder of cumin seeds' and 2 gms. of black salt. Grind them together to make it come in a homogeneous powder form. Add to it even amount of the kernel of the wood-apple. Mix the combination in about 100 gms. of curd to reactivate the sluggish liver. For early relief from any sort of stomach disorder, drink a spoonful of the combination of the juices of the basil and ginger.

Stones

Make the patient sit on a chair having a commod like opening on the seat. Now prepare the Karha of the blossoms of Basil, i.e., boil about 100 gms. of Basil blossom in a kilo of water. When the vapours start emerging, bring the container and stove beneath the chair on which the patient is seated. The moment the vapour starts touching the private organs, it would dissolve the stone. Continue this treatment for about a week for total cure.

T.B.

Grind together 5 grains of black pepper and 5 leaves of Basil leaves . Then mix the combination with half a spoonful of honey and lick it. Make the patient lick this combination twice daily. If it be winter season , add a little of ginger juice ,the husk of wheat and a little of salt also in the combination. This is a very effective treatment but it has to continue quite long. Externally, rubbing a little of Basil juice and ginger juice's mixture over the lungs shall bring the desired relief. Continue the treatment for about two months. Continue antitubercular treatment too.

Testcs Problem

If there be swelling on the testes or any other problem concerning with testes, apply the paste prepared in the following manner over the testes. Take about 5 gms. each of a camel's dung. Amarbel (easily available in Mango groves), the leaves of Arhar and Basil-leaves. Grind them to a homogeneous paste in a little of cow's urine. When the paste is ready, apply it over the testes thickly. Allow it to dry and remove it in the morning. A week's treatment will cure all troubles connected with the testes.

Urinary Problems

For any sort of this trouble, soak about 5 to 7 gms. of Basil seeds overnight in water. In the morning grind these seeds in water, add a litttle of sugar to the combination to make it more tasty. Drink this combination early in the morning and also in the afternoon, i.e., twice a day. Soon you will have copious discharge of urine and all problems connected with the urinary tract shall vanish in a week's time. Continue drinking raw milk and water mixture at least twice a day also.

Venereal Diseases (Male)

Basil leaves juice is very effective to cure all sort of these troubles. Take 5 gms. each of Basil seeds or dried Basil leaves and 5 gms. of tamarind. Now adding a little of honey to the combination make small tablets. These astringent tasting tablets should be taken at least four times a day. Don't swallow these tablets but suck it slowly.

If the accompanying cough be of dry type add a little of honey then additionally, make the patient have the combined juice extracted from the even amount of Basil seeds, ginger and onion. In case of wet-cough add sugar candy also in the combination.

Worms in Ears

If an insect be gone inside the ear or if there be worms in the ear or ears, in either case dropping a few drops of lukewarm Basil juice will provide immediate relief. If there be swelling in the ears, then add the juice of Bhangra with the juice of black Basil and put a few drops of this juice inside the affected or both the ears for quick relief.

Acidity

Take the dried blossom of Basil, rind of the Neem tree, black-pepper and peepal in even quantity and grind them to powder form. Take 3 gms. of this powder every morning and evening with plain water. All the acidic effect of the body shall pass out with urine and sweat. But remember, never to take milk over Basil leaves which might afflict your skin.

Black Spots

These are caused by excessive indulgence in the sexual pleasures which sap your vitality and these black spots appear. Extract a little of juice of Basil and add two times more lime juice. Make their homogeneous solution and apply this solution or paste over these spots every night with soft hands. The spots will be removed in a week's time. But restrain your sexual urges.

13

Home Treatment by Margosa

Margosa's properties are accepted worldwide and it has been patented also for it's medicinal properties.

Baldness

Applying Margosa oil on the bald position preferably at night and washing the head in the morning stops the failing of other hair and helps in their growth.

Falling of Hair and Greying Hair

(i) Washing the hair with water (in which Margosa and Berl or simple Margosa leaves are boiled) stops falling of hair and helps the hair to grow and be black and lustrous.

This is also useful to kill lices in the hair (Precaution this water should not entire the eyes).

(ii) Applying paste of leaves of Berl and Margosa In proportion of 2 :1 on the head and washing after 6-8 hrs. stops hair falling and makes them soft and shining.

(iii) Applying Margosa Tel helps in stopping fall and greying of hair and makes them black and soft. (Grind Margosa leaves with water and strain it. Mix sarson ka tel and extracted juice of Margosa in equal quantity and boil fton slow fire till all the water evaporates. After cooling store in a bottle for use).

(iv) Applying paste of nimbolis of Margosa and washing the head after 3-4 hours helps in eliminating lices and improves growth of hair.

Ear Trouble

Taking the steam of boiled water having Margosa leaves in it by the ear gives relief in ear-ache.

Dental Troubles

(i) Using fresh Margosa twig piece as brush for cleaning the teeth makes the gums strong, eliminates foul smell and cures pyorrhoea.

(ii) Use of Margosa tooth powder (Dry the branch of Margosa tree with leaves in shade burn it. Grind it with little pepperment, salt and cloves and then strain it through a cloth) strengthens the gums and teeth and checks foul smell.

(iii) Drinking and gargling with Margosa water (in which fresh new leaves are boiled) stops dental decay and pain in the teeth.

(iv) Gargling with margosa decoction (made with boiling of margosa leaves, flower, nimboli, root and branchs in equal proportion) gives relief to tooth-ache by eliminating infection in gums.

Cough

Gargles with Margosa juice mixed with few lukewarm drops of honey cures cough trouble.

Constipation

Rinsing the mouth with hot water in which 10 gms margosa leaves have been dissolved early in the morning cures constipation.

Vomiting

(i) Taking Margosa water (Grind 25 gms Margosa leaves mix it in 125 gm water and strain it) cures nausea and vomiting.

(ii) Applying paste of Margosa flower ground with water on the navel poition-stops vomiting.

Digestive Problems

Eating 10 fully ripe nimbolis daily with or after meals helps in curing indigestion.

Diarrhoea

(i) Heat inner bark of Margosa tree on iron tava. Grind it nicely when burnt, taking a pinch of this powder with curd helps in curing loose motions.

(ii) Swallowing powdered Margosa seed and sugar with water controls loose motions.

(iii) Taking ground 10 leaves of Margosa and Mishri with water checks diarrhoea especially in summers.

Dysentery

(i) Taking Margosa decotion (prepared by boiling margosa rind in double quantity of water) or 2 gm ground rind powder with water or honey juice in a day activates the system and controls dysentery.

(ii) Taking 10 gms. margosa juice of leaves in the morning also helps in curing it.

(iii) Taking decotion of Margosa leaves (Heat the juice of Margosa leaves on fire Cool and strain it) cures dysentery.

Fatigue

(i) Chewing a few margosa leaves helps in eliminating fatigue.

(ii) Eating chutney of Margosa leaves with little honey in it imparts energy and removes fatigue.

(iii) Chewing 5 leaves of Basil and 5 leaves of Margosa with honey gives instant relief and energy.

Itching and other skin ailments

(i) Applying paste of Nimbolis ground with water or Margosa oil on affected part cures itching.

(ii) Taking 20 gms of juice of soft fresh Margosa leaves 2 or 3 times a day cures itching caused by impurity of blood.

(iii) Taking 30 gm of Margosa juice (Soak ground Margosa leaves and flower if available in water overnight and strain it) with honey cures all impurities of blood.

(iv) Applying paste of Margosa leaves mixed with curd on affected part cures ring worm.

(v) Applying the Margosa ointment (put a branch with green leaves in boiling mustard oil in an iron utensil. Move it with Margosa stick until it gets thickened into ointment) on the affected part is very beneficial for all types of boils, pustules.

(vi) Taking 10 gms of Margosa tody (a type of secretion from certain Neern trees) cures all types of blood-impurities and checks skin diseases.

(vii) Taking this Margosa tody regularly for 6 months to 1 year is very helpful in chronic cases of leprosy and other skin diseases.

(viii) Taking 5 gm juice of fresh Margosa leaves and bathing with Margosa water (water with Margosa leaves boiled in it) helps in curing various skin diseases.

(ix) Swallowing 1 tsp powder of dried Margosa leaves, Margosa flower and Nimboli in equal quantity once in a day cures leucoderma.

(x) Taking fresh juice of Margosa leaves regularly stops the pimples and acnes. Applying paste of Margosa rind or Margosa oil also cures pimples and acnes.

Digestive and stomach ailments

(i) Taking 10 gms of powder (made by grinding rind of Margosa, dry ginger and black pepper-straining it through a fine cloth) with water in morning for 3 days cures acidity problem.

(ii) Taking ground 20 Margosa leaves, 2 cloves, 3 seeds of black pepper with little sugar and water twice a day for 2 to 3 days cures indigestion.

(iii) Eating 10-12 ripe nimbolis daily with or after food activates digestive system and normal appetite is resumed. This cures flatulence.

(iv) Taking 3 gms of margosa juice in ginger and mint juice 1gm each, little ajwain and kaala namak and sendha namak after food cures digestive problems.

(v) Drinking Margosa water (boil 100 gms of Margosa leaves in 250 gms water and strain it) 2 or 3 times a day helps in regaining normal appetite.

(vi) Taking 4 gms of churna (by grinding green but dry leaves) with water 3 or 4 times a day activates appetite and cures dyspesia.

Stones in Urinary Bladder

Taking 2 gm burnt ashes of Margosa leaves with water breaks the stones, which come out with urine. (Burn the leaves in a utensil after drying them in shade. Cover the utensil. After 4 hrs. grind the leaves).

Piles

(i) Taking 3-4 Nimbolis regularly helps in stopping excessive bleeding in piles.

(ii) Taking powder made of 3 gm inside part of the rind of margosa with 5 gm of jaggery regularly cures piles.

(iii) Applying and rubbing about 5 drops of Margosa oil on the haemorrhoids for 7-8 days helps in curing piles.

(iv) Taking powder of 10 Nimboli seeds, little sendha namak, gur jaggery or mishri with fresh water two times a day helps in curing piles.

Leucorrhoea

(i) Taking the juice of the rind of Margosa with white curninseeds checks leucorrhoea.

(ii) Drinking cow's milk with little Margosa oil in it at night regularly cures this.

Menstrual Disorders

(i) Taking juice of 10 fresh Margosa leaves and ginger juice in the same proportion with 10 gms water eliminates and cures excessive pain during menses.

(ii) Taking paste of Margosa leaves (Margosa leaves to be boiled and ground) below the navel will check pain during menses.

Labour Pains and Delivery

(i) Applying Margosa root in the waist of pregnant woman helps in early child birth (caution—this margosa root, should be thrown away soon after the child is born).

(ii) Taking Margosa water (in which Margosa leaves have been boiled for 15-20 minutes) will make the delivery less painful.

(iii) Taking juice of fresh, Margosa leaves on the 1st day of child-birth helps in contraction of uterus and works as an antiseptic.

(iv) Taking Margosa water (water in which Margosa bark is boiled) when thirsty for the 1st 6 days after child birth is good for the mother's health.

Urinary Problems

(i) Taking 15 gm juice of tender branches of Margosa with sharbat of unnab or sandalwood twice a day eliminates burning sensation or obstruction in the urinary passage.

(ii) Taking about 20-30 gms of juiceof root if sweet Margosa regularly cures urinary obstruction and burning.

Malaria

(i) Taking ground 2-3 leaves of Margosa with black pepper on the day of the turn of Malaria helps in checking it.

(ii) Taking 1 gm powder of dried Margosa leaves and posat boda. with water, checks the inset of fever (on its tumday).

(iii) Taking 60 gms ground margosa leaves, 4-5 black pepper seeds mixed with 120 gms of water twice a day works as a preventive against Malaria.

(iv) Massaging the scalp and hair with Margosa oil is also helpful.

Chronic Fever

Taking Margosa water (boil 500 gm water with 21 Margosa leaves and 21 black pepper seeds till the water is 125 gm) twice a day cures chronic fever.

Arthritis

(i) Massaging the swollen parts and other joints with Margosa oil is very useful. (Boil 50 gm mustard oil and put fresh margosa leaves in it till it become a bit black strain it and keep it in bottle). Even cooking the food in this Margosa oil is advisable for patients of Arthritis.

Paralysis

Massaging the affected protion with oil extraced from the seeds of Margosa invigorates the dead muscles and tissues.

Diabetes

Taking decoction of rind of Margosa (40 gms of the rind of margosa to be boiled in 100 gm. water till 30 gm. is left strain it) in the morning before breakfast eliminates sugar count in the urine.

Jaundice

(i) Taking 10 gms ground Margosa leave, 4-5 black pepper seeds and sugar with water in the morning regularly helps in eliminating the disease.

(ii) Taking ground Margosa leaves and sugar mixed with water after heating it a little cures the disease.

Asthma

Taking 25-30 drops of oil extracted from seeds of Margosa in bettle leaf gives great relief in Asthma.

Blister in the Mouth

Applying Margosa tel on the blisters with cotton cures them.

Sore Throat

Gargling with lukewarm juice of Margosa leaves and water cures soreness of the throat. 5 drops of honey and 2 drops of ginger juice may be added to extract the phlegm and eliminate the infection.

Heart Ailments

(i) Taking 10 gms juice of Margosa leaves, ground cumin-seeds, mint and kaala namak twice a day with lots of water intake during the day eliminates the burning sensation around the heart region.

(ii) Taking Margosa chutney with meals is very useful for controlling bile and stopping burning sensation.

(iii) Taking 1 tsp. of ground seeds of bakayan tree twice a day with water strengthens heart muscles and dissolves cholestrol.

Nose Bleeding

(i) Applying paste of Margosa leaves with little Ajwain on the temple stops bleeding.

(ii) Drinking juice of Margosa leaves like namkeen sharbat especially in summer is a preventive to those who suffer from nose-bleeding.

Poisonous Insect Bite

Chewing fresh Margosa leaves with or without little salt and pepper helps in eliminating poison.

Worms

(1) Giving 3-4 drops of Margosa tel to children and 5 to 6 drops to adults helps in killing the worms in intestines.

(ii) Taking 2 tsp fresh Margosa leaves juice with 1 tsp honey kills the worms.

(iii) Taking the paste of 1 tsp of juice of fresh Margosa leaves with a little heeng in it kills the worms.

Headache

Dropping one or two drops of juice of fresh Margosa leaves in the nostrils cures headache.

14

Home Treatment by Honey

Pure honey cures at least eighty ailments. It should be kept in every house.

Sterilization of Honey

One of the main objections to using honey has been that it may introduce a new infection from bacteria or spores present in the honey. Although it is generally thought that honey is a sterile product, bacteria and spores are able to survive in the honey but it is unlikely that they will actually grow in it unless the water content is too high. One report has shown that disease causing bacteria introduced into honey samples were capable of surviving 1.5 months to 2.4 years at 214F. Heat treatment or filtration through microporous membranes which are capable of preventing the passage of bacteria and spores are the usual ways medical products are sterilized. Sterilization of honey by heat treatment is not suitable because any hydrogen peroxide activity would be lost, and although it is more heat stable, there is also a reduction in the non-peroxide activity of Manuka honey at the temperatures required to ensure complete sterilization of honey. Filtration is also not suitable because of the high viscosity of honey, and particles present in the honey which block up the pores in the membranes. Gamma-irradiation, which is used to sterilize items such as surgical gloves and dressings which cannot be heat sterilized, was suggested as a possible alternative for sterilizing honey for use in hospitals. It may also be worth considering as an alternative to heat treatment of honey which is required when exporting to the Australian market. To determine whether this would have any effect on the antibacterial activity of the honey, samples were tested for activity before and after gamma-irradiation. The results showed that there was no significant reduction in the antibacterial activity of honeys containing hydrogen peroxide activity and Manuka honeys with non-peroxide activity.

Clinical Trial on Wound Healing

In conjunction with staff at Waikato Hospital a clinical trial is in its preliminary stages using honey as a wound dressing. The aim is to compare the effectiveness of honeys with the two different types of activity (hydrogen peroxide, and the non-peroxide activity of Manuka honey) and also compare these with a standard treatment. So far only Manuka honey has been used, and good results are being obtained.

Honey for the Treatment of Gastroenteritis

Currently, with funding by the Honey Industry Trust, a study is being carried out to determine whether organisms which cause gastroenteritis (diarrhea and vomiting), are sensitive to the peroxide and non-peroxide antibacterial activity of honeys. Again many reports have indicated that honey is an effective remedy for stomach upsets. One report in the British Medical Journal suggested that it shortened the duration of bacterial diarrhea and was as effective as glucose at promoting the re-absorption of sodium and water from the intestines.

As the major problem with gastroenteritis is that the patient becomes dehydrated, dosing with honey would help to replace lost electrolytes and provide an energy source as well.

A pasture blend honey with a high hydrogen peroxide activity and a Manuka honey with a medium non-peroxide activity are being compared with an artificial honey (a mixture of sugars at an acid pH similar to that found in honey). The artificial honey is used as a control to determine whether the antibacterial activity is due solely to the high sugar and low pH of honey or to some other factors present only in the honeys.

The results show that the organisms tested so far are inhibited by concentrations of 5-8% pasture blend (high peroxide) and 7-11% Manuka honey but it requires 20-30% artificial honey to have the same effect, clearly showing that factors other than sugar and pH are providing the antibacterial activity.

Although the bacteria tested so far have been isolated from human infections the indications are that honey could be equally effective and valuable as a remedy for scours in young animals such as calves.

It could also be used as an organic alternative to the antibiotic food supplement currently used for other animals including piglets and poultry. This avoids the problem of antibiotic residues. Bacteria isolated from animal sources will be tested in the next stage of the study.

Effect of Honey on Fungi

Another project recently funded by the Honey Industry Trust was to determine whether honey had any activity against a range of dermatophytes, i.e. fungi causing skin infections such as ringworm and athletes foot. All the fungi species tested were inhibited by low concentrations of the hydrogen peroxide activity but considerably higher concentrations of Manuka type non-peroxide activity were necessary for inhibition.

Precautions

DO NOT add honey to your baby's food, water or formula.

DO NOT dip your baby's pacifier in honey.

DO NOT give your baby honey as medicine.

Honey may contain Clostridium botulinum spores that can cause infant botulism—a rare but serious disease that affects the nervous system of young babies (under one year of age) C. botulinum spores are present throughout the environment and may be found in dust, soil and improperly canned foods. Adults and children over one year of age are routinely exposed to, but not normally affected by, C. botulinum spores.

Stomach Ulcers

In the traditional medicine of some parts of the world honey has also been used to treat dyspepsia and stomach ulcers. There are numerous reports of this treatment being used successfully in clinics in Russia in modern times, and a recent report of a clinical trial in Egypt which established that this traditional remedy is in fact effective.

However, there has been no explanation of how honey works in this treatment, which has prevented the treatment from being considered seriously by many in the medical profession.

In the last few years it has been recognized that dyspepsia and stomach ulcers are frequently caused by infection of the stomach by a species of bacteria, helicobacter pylori. The possibility that the healing effect of honey on the stomach may be through its acting on this bacterium was suggested by Niaz Al Somai at the University of Waikato. In collaboration with microbiologists at the Waikato Hospital he tested strains of helicobacter pylori isolated from biopsy samples of stomach ulcers, using the, same two honeys that had been tested on the wound-infecting species of bacteria. It was found that the honey with hydrogen peroxide activity did not prevent the growth of cultures of helicobacter pylori when added at concentrations up to 50%, but the Manuka honey completely halted growth of the bacterium at a concentration of 5%. A clinical trial was organized to find out if Manuka honey has the same effect on the bacterium in the stomach as it does when they are on agar plates. There is much interest in this possibility because conventional therapy for stomach ulcers is far from satisfactory. Drugs which prevent secretion of acid in the stomach may allow an ulcer to heal but it frequently re-appears. Only if helicobacter pylori is eliminated is a lasting cure achieved, but it is a very difficult infection to clear. A combination of antibiotics and bismuth is required, and unpleasant side-effects often result.

There is also the consideration that a very large amount of money is spent on the pharmaceuticals currently used to treat stomach ulcers. If honey is shown by clinical trial to be a reasonable alternative it would be a much cheaper option. The trial was abandoned without completion because the gastroenter-ologists were not entering sufficient patients, so no conclusive results were obtained regarding the ability of the treatment with Manuka honey to clear the bacterial infection. However, there was a clear indication that the patients taking the honey with antibacterial activity had significant relief from the discomfort and pain associated with their illness, whereas the patients taking honey without antibacterial activity did not. (Neither group of patients knew whether they were taking active or inactive Manuka honey, nor did their gastroenterologists know. The dosage used was 3/4 oz of honey four times a day, 1 hour before meals or at bedtime.)

Update on Current Research

This presentation is to provide an update on the current research into the antibacterial activity of honey being carried out at Waikato

University under the direction of Dr. Peter Molan. A priority at the present time is to provide scientific evidence of the effectiveness and safety of using honey as an alternative to conventional forms of treatment for skin and gastro-intestinal infections in the medical field and mastitis, wounds and scours in the veterinary fields. We have numerous reports, both scientific papers and personal communic ations, of honey being used successfully to treat ulcers, bedsores, wounds, burns, and dermatitis which were not responding to usual methods of treatment, but it has proven difficult to convince those in the medical and veterinary professions that honey is a safe effective remedy to use.

15

Home Treatment by Bangal Kins (Bael)

The ripe-fruit is nutritious, delicious, aromatic and laxative and both ripe and up-ripe fruit is used for curing many ailments.

CURATIVE PROPERTIES

Teething

Boil 10 gms powdered dried pulp of Bael fruit in 100 gms. water till the quantity of water is 20 gms.

5 gms of this mixed with little honey administered thrice a day for 3 days helps in teething.

Diarrhoea and Dysentary

(i) Pulp of unripe Bael with chacha (whey) controls diarrhoea.

(ii) Pulp of ripe Bael with water checks diarrhoea.

(iii) Preparation made by boiling pulp of unripe or half ripe Bael fruit acts an anti-flatulent and controls acidity, diarrhoea and dysentery.

(iv) Murabba of Bael also helps in controlling Diarrhoea and dysentery.

(v) Decoction of unripe Bael fruit baked for 6 hrs. with mishri controls dysentery.

Dyspepsia

Syrup of ripe fruit helps in dyspepsia.

Piles

Pulp of ripe fruit mixed with mishri checks constipation and controls piles.

Vomiting

(i) Decoction of unripe Bael fruit controls vomiting.

(ii) Pulp of ripe fruit (20 gms) mixed with water of boiled rice and little mishri controls vomiting during pregnancy.

Anaemia

(i) 5 gms powder of dried pulp mixed with milk and little sugar checks anaemia.

(ii) Powder of dried pulp with Chacha with little sugar eliminates blood impurities.

Leucorrhoea

Make powder of 10 gm pulp of Bael, mixed with 10 gm Nagkesar and 10 gm-Rasont. 5 gms of this mixture taken with Maand (boiled-rice water) checks leucorrhoea.

Cholera

50 gms juice of leaves mixed with little lemon-juice and desi khand taken daily prevents Cholera.

Whooping Cough

Roast the green leaves on slow fire till they become black powder. Filter them through cloth, 1 or 2 gms of this powder taken with little honey 3 times a day checks whooping cough.

Kanthamala

Make a paste of fresh leaves mixed with pure ghee. Apply the paste twice a day around the neck and cover with a cloth. It helps in eliminated Kanthamala.

Night blindness (Nyctalopia)

Grind 10 gms fresh leaves and 7 seeds of black pepper with little water and mix it with 25 gms of sugar in 100 gms water. Taking this twice a day helps in night-blindness.

Also soak a few.leaves in water overnight and wash the eyes with that in the morning.

Bronchitis

Poultice prepared from the leaves is applied to the chest in acute bronchitis.

Asthma

A decoction of leaves of Bael helps in asthma.

Diabetes

(i) Juice of bael leaves with ground black pepper is useful in Diabetes.

(ii) Chewing 4-6 Bael-leaves daily controls sugar.

Urinary Irritation

Juice of bael leaves, ground jeera and mishri (all in equal quantity) taken with milk stops urinary irritation.

Repellant of Mosquitoes and Insects

Burning of outershell of the Bael repels all insects and mosquitos.

Thus the Bael tree is very significant. Apart from nutritional and medicinal value of the ripe, and unripe fruit pulp, the other parts of the tree its bark, flowers, leaves, trunk etc. have their special properties and uses. Bael is widely used as a medicine in households.

16

Home Treatment by Banana

Banana is a fruit with lots of medicinal value. It is a good source of calcium and fibre.

Constipation and Diarrhoea

Bananas are of great value both in constipation and diarrhoea as they normalise colonic functions in the large intestine to absorb large amounts of water for proper bowel movements. Their usefulness in constipation is due to their richness in pectin, which is water-absorbent and this gives them a bulk producing ability. They also possess the ability to change the bacteria in the intestines-from the harmful type of bacilli to the beneficial acidophyllus bacilli.

Intestinal Disorder

Banana is used as a dietary food against intestinal disorders because of its soft texture and blandness. It is said to contain an unidentified compound called, perhaps jointly, vitamin U' (against ulcer). It is the only raw fruit which can be eaten without distress in chronic ulcer. It neutralises the over-acidity of the gastric juices and reduces the irritation of the ulcer by coating the lining of the stomach.

Ripe bananas are highly beneficial in the treatment of ulcerative colitiso being bland, smooth, easily-digestible and slightly laxative. They relieve acute symptoms and promote the healing process.

Dysentery

Mashed banana together with little salt is a good remedy for dysentery. According to Dr. Kirticar, a combination of ripe plantain, tamarind and common salt is most effective in this disease. He claims to have cured several cases of both acute and chronic dysentery by this treatment. Ripe bananas are also very useful in dysentery of children, but they should be thoroughly mashed and beaten to cream before use in these cases

Arthritis and Gout

Bananas are useful in the treatment of arthritis and gout. A diet of bananas only for three or four days is advised in these conditions. The patient can be given to eat eight or nine bananas daily during this period and nothing else.

Anaemia

Being high in iron content, bananas are beneficial in the treatment of anaemia. They stimulate the production of haemoglobin in the blood.

Allergies

The fruit is very useful for those who are allergic to certain foods and who suffer in consequence from skin rashes or digestive disorders or asthma. Unlike other protein foods, many of which contain an amino-acid which these persons cannot tolerate and which causes allergy. Bananas contain only benign amino-acids which in most cases automat allergic. The fruit, however, does cause allergic reactions in certain sensitive persons and they should avoid it.

Kidney Disorders

Bananas are valuable in kidney disorders because of their protein and salt content and high carbohydrate content. They are useful in uraemia, a toxic condition of the blood due to kidney congestion and dysfunction. In such cases, a diet of bananas should only be taken for three to four days, consuming eight to nine bananas a day. This diet is suitable for all kidney troubles, including nepthritis.

Tuberculosis

Bananas are considered useful in the treatment of tuberculosis. According to Dr. J. Montelvz of Brazil, South America, the juice of the plantain or the ordinary cooked bananas works miracles in the cure of tuberculosis. He claims to have cured patients with advanced stage of tuberculosis with frequent cough, abundant expectoration or phlegm and high fever in two months by this treatment.

Urinary Disorders

Juice from banana stem is a well-known remedy in urinary disorders. It improves the functional efficiency of kidney and liver thereby alleviating the discomforts and diseased condition in them. It clears the excretionory organs in the abdominal region of toxins and helps to eliminate them in the form of urine. It has been found to be of great help in the treatment for the removal of stones in the kidney, gall bladder, and prostate. It is advisable to mix this juice whenever possible with the juice of ash pumpkin.

Over-weight

A diet consisting of bananas and skimmed milk is considered an effective remedy for weight reduction. In prescribed course of diet treatment, the daily diet is restricted to six bananas and four glasses of skimmed milk or buttermilk made from skimmed milk for a period of 10 to 15 days. Thereafter green vegetables may be introduced gradually, reducing the intake of bananas from six to four. This regimen for, prescribed course of diet treatment can be continued till the desired results are achieved. Bananas are suitable for overweight people as they contain practically no sodium.

Menstrual Disorders

Cooked banana flower eaten with curd is considered an effective medicine for menstrual disorders like painful menstruation and excessive bleeding. Banana flower help increase progesterone hormone which reduces the bleeding.

Burns and Wounds

A plaster is prepared by beating a ripe banana into a fine, paste. It can be spread over burns and wounds and supported by a cloth bandage. It gives immediate relief. The young tender leaves of banana tree form a cool dressing for inflammation and blisters.

Uses

Ripe bananas are chiefly eaten raw as a dessert or a breakfast fruit. It is also used in salad together with other fruits and vegetables. Unripe fruits are cooked. Banana chips are made from fully mature unripe fruits. The flour prepared from the dried unripe bananas is three times richer in minerals than the wheat. It is more digestile than cereal starches and is an ideal food for infants and invalids.

Precautions

Banana, taken as a table fruit, must be thoroughly ripe as otherwise it may be difficult to digest. The raw bananas contain 20 to 25 per cent starch. But during the process of ripening, this: starch is almost wholly converted with assimilable sugar.

Bananas should never be kept in a refrigerator as low temperature prevents their ripening. The fruit should not be taken by those who are suffering from kidney failure because of its high potassium content.

17

Home Treatment by Date

Dates are valuable as medicine for their tonic effect. Being easily digested, they are very useful for supplying energy and repairing waste. Milk in which clean and fresh dates have been boiled is a very nourishing and restorative drink to children and adults alike, especially during convalescence.

Constipation

The date is a laxative food. It is highly beneficial in the treatment of constipation as the roughage provided by it stimulates sluggish bowels. They should be immersed in water at night and taken after making them into a fine syrup the next morning to secure laxative effect.

Intoxication

Dates are an excellent remedy for alcoholic intoxication. In such cases, drinking water in which fresh dates have been rubbed or soaked will bring quick relief.

Intestinal Disturbances

The nicotinic content in dates is an excellent remedy for intestinal disturbances. According to Metchnikoff, the great Russian scientist, liberal use of dates keeps in check the growth of pathological organisms and helps to establish a colony of friendly bacteria in the intestines.

Weak Heart

Dates are an effective remedy for weak heart. Dates soaked overnight in water and crushed in the same water in the morning after removing the seeds should be taken at least twice a week in this condition. It will strengthen the heart.

Sexual Debility

Dates are highly beneficial in the treatment of sexual weakness. A handful of dates soaked in fresh goat's milk overnight should be ground in the same milk in the morning. A pinch of cardamom powder and honey should be mixed in this preparation. This becomes a very useful tonic for improving sex stamina and sterility due to functional disorders.

Children's Diseases

According to Dr. Aman, a date tied to the wrist of the baby and allowed to be sucked by him during teething time hardens the gums and prevents other complaints like fretfulness and diarrhoea. A teaspoonful of paste of the date prepared with honey is an effective medicine for diarrhoea and dysentery during teething. It should be given three times a day.

Precautions

The dates require great care for selection. The sticky surface of the date attracts dust and impurities of the air to settle there. It is, therefore, advisable to purchase the best varieties in good packing condition and to wash them thoroughly before use.

18

Home Treatment by Fruits

Anaemia

There are many fruits and flowers which offer permanent cure for the patient

(i) Give the patient half a kg. of sweet grapes' juice for 10 days. He shall have enough blood in the body with rich haemoglobin in it.

(ii) Have (Peaches) Aaddoos at least 5 at a time for about 10 days. Peaches are rich in iron and they would cure this trouble.

(iii) Suck about 200 gms. of Falsey every day. If you like you can chew them also.

(iv) Have mango - juice and milk combination for about a week.

Baldness

Take the oil of the mango pickle and massage your skull for about half an hour with it. If you are bald not because of the hereditary effect, you would definitely get back your hair. During the season of kakadis (cucumber) crush them and extract their juice and apply it on your hair for a fortnight. You can also apply their pulp on your head for quick hair-growth.

Bed Wetting

Feed such children on dry dates (Chhuhare) pieces before they go to sleep. Don't let them have tea when it is dark. Give them Halwa of potatoes instead. The most effective treatment for such chronic patients is to give them about 2 gms. of the powdered stone of Jamun with water. In a couple of days this problem will be solved for ever.

Blood Impurity

Shahtoot has this admirable quality to cure all the impurities of blood. Just take about 250 gms. of Shahtoot early in the morning instead of your normal breakfast and follow it up by the even quantity of Shahtoot in the evening also. These two doses will cure the blood totally.

Bronchitis

Take about 10 almonds and 10 dried raisins (Munnakka) and soak them in water overnight. Early in the morning remove the rinds from Badam (almonds) and unseed the raisins. Now take a small, cleaned piece of ginger and grind the three ingredients to a paste form. Now add two spoons of honey and lick it. Do it every evening and morning for two days. This treatment will not only cure the trouble but would also strengthen your lungs.

Burning in Urethra

First, try to ascertain the cause of this burning. If it is caused by the unhygienic condition of the area, clean it by lukewarm water. If it is caused by eating lots of chillies, stop eating them. Always drink a lot of water half an hour after having your meals. If it is being caused by some inside problem, extract the juice of the fresh Amla, add a little of sugar candy and drink it thrice a day. In just three days' time this trouble will be cured. Amla will cleanse the renal region which is causing the burning and then this problem shall be over. But always keep the area clean.

Cholera

First of all extract the juice of a couple of onions and give it to the patient. Then prepare the lemon syrup and ask the afflicted person to drink it slowly by gradually sipping it. If still the patient be feeling nausea, then feed him again on the onion juice. Add a little of lemon juice and black-pepper, rock salt also in the onion juice.

This dose will definitely cure the trouble. But keep on making the patient drink lots of water. O.R.S. powder is available an every medical store, which can be of great help in curing cholera.

Contipation

(i) Take about two spoonfuls of gulkand and drink a glass of lukewarm milk in the night, over it. Next day you will have clear motion.

(ii) Have mangoes and then drink a glass of hot water over it for curing the trouble.

(iii) Have half a cup of peaches juice for quick cure of the constipation.

(iv) Howsoever chronic be your constipation, if you take a glass of diluted orange juice on empty stomach after brushing your teeth, you'll never have this problem.

If cough be of dry type (having no expectoration of phlegm), then take the kernal of the mango-stone, reduce it to powdered form and lick it at least twice or thrice every day till fully cured.

In case the cough be with phlegm expectoration, take the rind of a pomegranate and keep on licking it. Alternatively, extract the juice of ripe apples and drink at least half a glass of it every morning and evening for complete cure. Having ginger and boil leaves and boil leaves juice mixed with honey shall also help.

Chronic Wound

Bring a piece of mango bark and boil it in water to make its thick paste. When the paste cools down a bit, apply daily on the wound. This paste is anti-septic and full of healing qualities. The best way to apply it is to take it on a soft cloth or cotton, put it over the wound. Do it every evening and morning. In three or four applications the wound would heal up. If the wound be quite deep, it might take longer time for the new flesh to appear. Keep the wound clean by washing it with warm water. In homoeopathy a drug colemdula is made from Genda flowers, which is a great antiseptic.

Diabetes

Extract half a cup of Jamun juice and add equal amount of Karela juice. Mix then drink the mixed juice as the first thing in the morning. In about a fortnight the miraculous effect can be seen. Together with it, grind the stone of Jamun to powder form and keep it in a clean bottle. Take this powder daily only half a spoonful every morning and evening with water. These remedies shall not only help cure diabetes but will also help check the onset of diabetes. In about three months time the total relief could be expected.

Dysentery

Take about 10 gms. each of the kernal of jamun and mango stones and grind them to powdered form. Mix about 2 gms. of this mixture of the powder in 100 gms. of curd and eat it. Do so at least twice a day, preferably after breakfast and lunch. In summers you can also take it during the night. This regular intake will cure the trouble in about a week's time. But such persons must not ocnsume fried and fat rich items and should start taking a long walk in the morning.

Drug Intoxication

If the person is having Bhang or opium intoxication, then treat the afflicted person in the following way:

(i) Ask the patient to take a Guava and allow him to sleep. The intoxication will be cured.

(ii) If it is not be guava season, you can have a few soft leaves (10-15) of guava, grind them and extract their juice. Give it to the patient for drinking.

(iii) To kill the heat of the intoxication, extract a little juice of tamarind and give it to the person for drinking. This will quickly cure the intoxication.

(iv) Ask the patient to lick the Lemon. This is also helpful in curing bad effects of intoxication.

Eczema

Normally we throw away the thick covering of the water-melon (Tarbooz). If we burn it and keep the ash in a clean bottle, this is a very effective remedy for eczema. If eczema be of weeping type, just sprinkle a little of this ash for quick relief. If it be for dry type, add this ash to a little of mustard oil and apply it on the affected part. In about a week's time the skin will become soft and healthy. But don't touch tea or coffee for about a week.

Ear Boil

Collect a little of green blossom of mango normally lying beneath the mango tree. Extract the juice of this green blossom, add in even amount of mustard oil and put a few drops of it in the afflicted ear. This treatment will make the boil burst and clear out all the pus etc.

Early Aging

Take about 10 almonds, soak them in water, remove their rinds and grind them to paste from mixing a little of milk. Now boil the combination in milk and when cool, add about two spoonfuls of honey. Drink this portion like you are sucking it. Continue the treatment for about a year. Have lots of apples, grapes and oranges daily.

Extreme Thirst

Normally the thirst is easily quenched by drinking juices of orange, pineapple or caneapple. Still if you fail to quench the thirst then try the following remedy:

Take out the kernal from a mango-stone and crust it and boil it in water like you boil tea. Now add a little of sugar candy and drink it like you drink tea.

For those who frequently feel extremely thirsty, pomegranate juice mixed with sugarcandy is the ideal combination. Drink it twice or thrice to overcome this feeling.

Epileptic Attack

For those affiliated with epilepsy, phosphorus rich fruits are essential. If they continue to have the juice of shahtoot (25 gms only) daily, this divine juice will provide enough strength to the nerves to fight out this affliction. In the absence of shahtoot, the juice of ripe apples or sev ka murabba (Jam of Apple) should be given. Figs also help the nerves to acquire strength. Lightly roast figs on fire and allow the patient to eat it, and wash it down with the juice of ripe apples.

Fire Burns

If the fire-burn be not very deep, extract the kernal from the mango stone, rub it against water surface and apply the rubbed paste on the burns. Soon the cool relief will be felt. If it be a form of wound, burn the dry leaves of mango, strain the ash and sprinkle over the wound. This ash is antiseptic and very good to heal the fire burns.

Fatigue

Narial-Pani (coconut - water) immediately removes fatigue and brings energy back to the body. Having orange juice with little of pineapples juice mixed in it shall quickly remove the fatigue. While drinking these, rinse them in your mouth and keep you tongue standing clean of the teeth for quick rejuvenation.

Foul smell from Breath

Normally this foul breath is caused by not any infection in the mouth but due to digestive disorders. Take 5 grains of Munnakka (raisins) and 5 pieces of small cardamom. Remove the seeds of Munnakka and replace them by the grains of small cardamom. Lick their juice without chewing them. Soon your breath would become fresh.

Gout

Get the oil from the kernel of mango stone extracted and then use this oil in massaging the aching joints. This massage cures even the most chronic aching joints. Alernatively, have 125 gms. of 'Chaman Ka Angoor' (the grapes from CHAMAN), regularly in your breakfast for at least a fortnight for getting total relief from the trouble. Then after reducing the quantity of the grapes dose and enhance the intervening period. Grapes do not allow any raw phlegm to settle on joints.

Giddiness

Take 10 Munnakkas (raisins) and immerse them in a glassful of water. Keep the glass in such a position that solar rays strike direct at the portion of glass containing Munnakkas. This water heat will bloat up the Munnakkas. Now remove their seeds, chew the pulp of Munnakka and wash it down by water Munnakkas were soaked in. The giddiness will vanish.

Gonorrohoea

Take about a handful of the seeds of musk-melon (Kharbooza). Remove their covering to get to their kernal. Now rub them against stone to grind them to make their Sherbat. Add about 10 drops of Sandalwood oil to it. Ask the patient to have twice this sherbat. Continue the treatment for about 10 to 15 days or till this illness is totally cured.

Hair-loss

Sometimes malnutrition result in hair-loss. It means hair are not getting their due food and getting weak on their roots. Sometimes people who become habitual Bhang or Afeem (opium) addicts suffer from this problem. The hair get too dry owing to malnutrition. Having Jamun and applying coconut oil externally is the tired and tested remedy to stop hair-loss. To regain hair at the skull, apply pulp or juice of kakadi (cucumber) juice-massage it and leave as it is for half an hour before bath.

High Blood Pressure

Cut a huge Tarbooz (watermelon) separate its seeds and sprinkle rock-salt and a little of black pepper. Do so while keeping it in a big steel plate. Now give all the cut pieces of the melon to your friends and relations and have only seeped out tarbooz—water is a very good tonic because it contains minerals like phosphorus iron and vitamins in rich quality. Those who can, may avoid salt at all or have very little of sendha salt. This water is also a good tonic for nerves and nerves shall be relaxed also.

Heat Stroke

The juice of raw mangoes popularly known as 'Panna' is a very effective anti-dote of heat stroke. Lightly roast a raw mango and crush it to extract its juice, throwing away the rind and stone. Now, in this juice add a little of black-pepper powder, common rock salt and sugar. Just drink this juice and you shall not feel any adverse effect of heat. If one already is struck by heat, then applying pulp of tamarind over hand and feet will immediately lower the body temperature and the heat's effect will be neutralised.

Heart Ailment

Juice of Mausambi is ideal to reduce the cholesterol level in the blood whose increase causes all sorts of heart ailments. Besides clearing the excessive cholesterol, Mausambi juice also brings freshness to the system. But drink this juice without ice as ice dilutes its effect. This juice would keep heart vessels soft and supple and blood with have smooth circulation also.

Alternatively mix sugarcandy powder in the even amount of Amla powder and have it every morning and evening with water for quick cure of all sorts of heart ailments.

Indigestion

Cut a fresh Papaya, sprinkle rock salt and black-pepper over its pieces and pour few-drops of lemon and eat them gradually. Papaya has a very useful element 'Pepsin' which is very good to clear any sort of indigestion. Not only it clears indigestion, but also cures the germs inside the body. It is an ideal fruit to activate the sluggish liver. Besides cleaning infection and curing indigestion, Papaya also provides energy to the body.

Influenza

Take a Chakotara (botanical name Citrus Decumana) and cut it to small pieces. Then suck all these pieces one by one. Its juice is a very good antidote for the flu germs.

Alternatively, if a shaddock be not available, one can replace it by diluted orange juice. Extract the juice of 2-3 orange, add 1/4th water to it and sip this diluted juice twice or thrice a day. Having citrus fruits is helpful to cure flu because of the large quantity of Vitamin "C" in them.

Impotence

Take two Chhuhares (dried dates) and 10 raisins—boil them and grind them together. Now add to it the ground paste of 10 almonds after soaking them overnight and removing their skin. Now add a little of honey in the paste and add both the pastes together. Now eat a spoonful or two with a glass of hot milk. Although it can be eaten with dinner also, yet in many cases this combination causes night discharge. Hence it is better to have this combination with breakfast. In less than two weeks the trouble will vanish.

Jaundice

Jaundice results when we eat infected food items. Here the colour of body becomes yellow. Hence such a patient must be fed on those fruits and flowers which have these contents in adequate quantity. Having Dates, Peaches, aloobukhara, whey from unsour curd, red raisin (Munnakka) beetorrt, tomatoes, strawberry mixed with honey will eke out these elements and you would again start to have your blood red and healthy. And jaundice shall automatically be taken care of.

Kidney - pain

Having the decoction (porha) of the leaves of grapes quickly cures this trouble. Boil about 30 to 40 leaves of grapes in water, then add a little rock salt and strain it through a coarse cloth. Now allow the patient to drink it. While preparing the Karha take care that you use only soft leaves and boil them after thoroughly cleaning them. This Karha is very effective to cure all sort of kidney troubles.

Liver-trouble

Tomato juice and soup of tomato is very effective to activate a sluggish liver. Make the patient drink the juice early in the morning and soup in lunch or dinner. For elderly persons juice of two tomatoes and for younger patient, of one tomato would be adequate. Add a little of ginger juice with tomato juice to benefit the bowels also.

Alternatively collect the dried broken leaves of mango normally found lying beneath the mango tree. Boil these the same way you boil tea-leaves and drink them like you drink tea just once a week to keep you liver in good working.

Lices

Take the rind of pomegranate, dry it and then grind it to put the dried powder in a bottle. Whenever any one has this trouble, add this powder in water to form a paste and apply this paste to hair. Keep it as it is and after half an hour of this application, wash it off. The lices will be cleared off the head. The powder of Sharifa seeds is also effective to clear lices.

Leucorhoea

Those ladies who are afflicted with this trouble must take the powder of the kernal of mango at least twice or thrice a day with water. Another good treatment is having the starchy fluid of the rice mixed in jamun juice. Another remedy is to hack of katira gond (gum) to small pieces, then soak them in water and have those bloated pieces of gond with milk.

Loss of Appetite

Many a time this loss of appetite results due to over-eating or eating very heavy food at irregular hour. In such a case, leaving food for a day or two is good proposition. If it is caused by some internal disturbance in the digestive system, then having 7 or 8 leeches would be best remedy. Do not eat them but gradually suck them. By the time you have licked the eight lichee your desire for food will increase. Having lemon-juice diluted in water is also very effective to restore your appetite.

Malaria

This dreadful infection is caused by the mosquitoes. First of all you must keep your area clear of any filth and dirt. Since the fever comes after a shuddering sensation, the patient should be well covered in quilts or blankets. Give the patient diluted juice of shaddock to drink. Shaddock or chakotara has the capacity to kill these germs.

Drinking chirayata solution is an age-old anti-dote of malaria. To lessen its bitterness you can add a little of orange juice. Juice of cinamon's bark is also useful.

Memory Loss

Leechi and apples are very effective to revive one's memory cells. Have your normal food followed by a glass of whey seasoned with as afoetida and cumin seeds. Stop drinking water with your meals. With lunch drink a glass of whey and after dinner a glass of cow's milk having a little of honey mixed in it. If you eat a lot of leeches and apples, your memory would definitely be revived in about a month or so. Keep your system clear of constipation.

Miscarriage

If there be no deficiency in the productive organs of the lady, then this problem can be successfully tackled with the help of the leaves of raspberry or rasbhari. Such ladies, immediately after conception must drink the concoction of the leaves of raspberry. Prepare the concoction like you prepare tea. And instead of adding the leaves of tea, put the leaves of raspberry in the milk-sugar solution. These leaves are quite rich in iron, phosphorus and calcium which are the necessary elements to develop the foetus.

Mouth Boils

Take a few soft leaves of guava. Extract their juice, add a little cachet (Katha) powder and apply this paste over the mouth boils. Then allow the saliva to ooze out. Soon the boils would start drying up. Alternatively, add a well ripe banana in sweet curd. Now gradually apply this solution with the help of a spoon. A couple of doses of this dish will clean the mouth boils in a few days.

Migraine

Those who have their houses located amidst the mango groves seldom suffer from this trouble. You must have seen parrots pecking up the mango blossom which lies scattered beneath the mango trees. Select a few bunches of green blossom and grind them to extract about half a spoonful of their juice. Put a few drops of this juice in the opposite nostril you are having pain in, or apply it by your finger over your nostril. Now lie down in a dark room. In just a couple of days this problem shall be taken care of and you shall be cured.

Nausea

Take a bit of aam ka papad and give it to the person suffering from this trouble. The feeling of nausea shall vanish soon.

Altertnatively, if it be the mango season, ask the person to suck mangoes which has a very thin juice. If mangoes be not available, take about 25 gms. of orange juice and add about two spoonfuls of honey. Now make the afflicted person drink it drop by drop. Soon the feeling of nausea shall vanish.

Nose Bleeding

Extract the juice of green mango kernal by adding a little of water. Just two drops would be quite sufficient. Put these drops in each nostril to stop nose-bleeding. Look at a very good fruit and its consumption stops nose bleeding almost immediately.

Night Blindness

As we all know the night blindness is caused by the lack of Vitamin "A" in the system. Such persons should consume mangoes, tomatoes, cabbage and honey. The more of these items are consumed the better would be you eye-sight in nights.

Night Discharge

Add a little of alum in the juice of mango and apply this solution around your penis during sleep. Although it might give a sticky feeling yet in about 10 to 12 days you shall be rid of this problem.

To thicken your semen take about 2 gms. of Jamun-stone's powder mixed in about 5 gms. of amla powder with honey. Continue both the treatments simultaneously and you shall be totally cured of this trouble. But stop reading pornographic books or seeing obsence movies.

Obstruction in the Urinary Passage

Just grind a few anwalas and apply the paste on and around penis and the lower stomach. You would have copious discharge of urine. Cucumber or kheera is a very good diuretic agent. Hack off their tops, remove their skin and eat them as much as you like. Sprinkel a bit of common slat and lemon for better taste. Soon you will feel the urge to urinate and all the obstruction will pass out with it. You can eat a lot of musk-melon for this purpose. All these watery fruits are very effective diuretic agents.

Pain in Knees

Strawberry is the ideal fruit to cure this trouble, since its chemical analysis revealed that after figs, the iron content is maximum in a strawberry fruit. It is equally rich in calcium. Have as much fresh strawberries as you like. You can always chew a few leaves of basil (Tulsi) for better result. Walking a lot and having strawberry are the necessary steps to cure this trouble permanently. Walk slowly but for a long distance.

Piles

For common type of Piles having the powdered form of the kernal of the mango-stones with whey is very effective. Take just 2.5 gms. of this powder with 100 gms. of whey. The haemorhoids will soon dry up. While continuing this treatment, smelling the blossom of mango will also help. For bleeding type, having Amla powder with whey is good. The proportion should be 3 gms. of the powder and 100 gms. whey. Figs are also very effective. Soak about 5 figs at a time in water and have them in the morning and evening for early cure.

Paralysis

Although there could be innumerable reasons of paralysis, yet if it is caused by clots in the brain or due to high blood pressure, the best is to feed the patient exclusively on apple, and grape juice. These juices are mixed in equal quantities and give to patients four times one up at a time. For external massage the best juice is that of a bottlegourd. Just extract this juice and rub it forcefully on the affected portion for relief. If it be winter season then dry fruits like almonds, cashew and pista could also be included in his diet. If one strictly adheres to this treatment then in about two months' time the cure can be possible.

Palpitation of Heart

If it be caused by some traumatic happening in the patient's life, washing of hands and feet will restore it to normal palpitation. If the cause be extreme heat, have just a couple of leeches or falsey or aloobukhara. Soon the palpitation will be normal. If it s a chronic trouble then having juice of ground pomegranate leaves can provide quick relief consult your physician as soon as possible.

Ricket

Add equal amount of grape juice in orange and ask the patient to drink the lot at least three times a day. Just 50 gms. of juice at a time will do.

If the child be having teeth, then give him dates to eat after dipping them in honey. Just five to six dates with honey a day will be enough to make the child grow well in a week's time. If the child be just a infant, give him the syrup of honey to drink. Mix two spoonfuls of honey in a cupful of water to prepare this syrup. If the child be in the feeding stage, the mother should apply honey on her nipples before feeding her child.

Sleep Walking

This is a very dangerous habit and can even prove fatal. Such persons should be fed exclusively on mango and milk combination or what is known as 'Amar Kalpa'. During this period the person is not given anything else but mango and milk. Mango-milk combination would energise nerves to cure this trouble.

Stone in Bladder

Normally the seeds of grapes, oranges or munnakkas (raisins) are thrown away because they create stone. But if the seeds of grapes are crushed and their powder's only half gm. quantity is taken with milk every evening, stones will be dissolved and thrown out of the system.

The juice of pears is also capable to dissolve the stones. The juice of slightly raw type of apples is also effective to do so. But it should be taken with adequate quantity of black pepper sprinkled over it.

Swelling in Spleen

Jamun is very effective to cure all the afflictions connected with spleen. Drink the juice of Jamun every day in the afternoon for curing the swelling in spleen.

Alternatively, during the mango season drink a glass of mango-shake after adding a little of honey. Continue this treatment for 21 days for total cure of this problem.

During the off season of mango or jamun, roast lightly a lemon and suck it after sprinkling rock salt and black pepper for about a week.

Tonsilitis

This is a very disturbing problem as the patient is unable to eat or drink properly. First of all, start the treatment by making the patient gargle with lukewarm water to which a little of alum has been added. After half an hour of this throat-cleaning process, drink half a glass of the juice of shahtoot (cane-apple). The juice is not only antiseptic but also has admirable healing powers. Since its ultimate effect on the body is cool, it also lessens the pain in the throat due to burning. Continue the treatment for a couple of days for total cure.

Testicle Swelling

Extract the kernal of the stones of leechi. Then lightly roast them over fire am grind them to paste form. Then apply it over the testicles while lukewarm. One or two applications will subside the swelling. If needed be you can repeat the remedy after a week or so.

Another very effective remedy is following: Take about two handfuls of mango leaves and add a little of salt to them. Now grind both of them. Add a little of water to make a thick paste, then heat it a little and apply over the testicles.

Teeth Troubles

(i) Collect the flowers of the pomegranate tree normally found lying beneath the tree. Dry them in the shade after cleaning them and then grind them to powdered form. Use this powder as tooth-powder. This is a very useful tooth-powder to stop blood oozing from the teeth, and also making teeth strong.

(ii) During the mango season, go to a mango grove early in the morning. Pluck a few of mango leaves, the soft ones— chew them repeatedly and then spit out the juice. Just in a week's time your teeth shall be firm and shining.

(iii) For those persons whose teeth have become disfigured because of eating too much of Pan Masala, etc. and have grown weak due to the effect of lime in the Pan Masala, the following tooth paste would be very good to keep the teeth firm and shining. Add a little of mustard oil in a spoonful of common salt and sprinkle a few drops of lemon juice over it. Daily rub your teeth with this paste to keep your teeth firm and sparkling.

Urinary Troubles

If the urine be persistently having deep yellow colour, it means that the tract is infected. Add a little of plain sugar in the syrup of canebeerry (Shahtoot) and drink it at 6 hourly interval for two days. The infection will be totally cured.

In case you have the problem of repeated urination, take about five to six Lisore (cordial maxi tree's fruits, also known as Labhere and chew them repeatedly. Soon the repeated urination problem will cured. If Labhere be not available, take about 2 to 3 gms. of the pomegranate rind's powder and swallow this powder with water. In a few hours you will feel the desired relief.

Veneral Diseases

Kharbooza or water-melon offers good treatment for these sort of diseases in which the heat of the body increases tremendously because of the infection. The juice of tarbooz is a good diuretic and through urine body heat is lessened in the body by taking it out of the body. Since all these diseases damage the body by creating heat, tarbooz (water melon) juice is a good remedy. The more the patient urinates, the earlier he should be cured. Alternatively add the cucumber juice in kalami shora (salt peter) and make the patient drink it twice a day for quick relief, But one should avoid having fried things, liquor, etc.

Weakness in General

For general tonic, Cheeku is the ideal fruit. Have about 6 or 8 Cheekus a day. Still better, if you have these Cheekus after breakfast and lunch and apple juice in the afternoon. Cheeku would provide the necessary strength and apple juice would fill the body up by flesh. But make sure that neither the cheekus nor the apples should be raw or overripe. In just a week's time your body would become powerful and glowing with pink health. But during the period you must tire yourself physically so that these juices provide the necessary fillip to the body.

Whopping Cough

Grate off the small bristles normally found on the stone of kalami mangoes. About a handful would be sufficient. Now burn these bristles to ashes form. When cool, preserve it in a bottle. Now, daily in the night take two gms. of this ash by mixing it with honey and give it to the patient for licking it after adding just a drop of garlic juice. This is tried and tested combination to clear the throat and chest congestion and cure this disease, which normally afflicts children.

Worms in Intestines

For getting rid of these worms, no need to eat fruits but their rinds. Although it might sound rather unusual, yet it is a tested remedy. Collect the rinds of pomegranates and oranges. Dry them and grind them. Now take just 2-3 grams of this rind powder, mix it in about

50 gms. of separated whey or chhach and add salt according to taste. Adding salt is essential as salt kills these worms easily. Have this dose twice or thrice a day. In a couple of days you would be cured of this disease. Having shahtoot (camelemy) is also beneficial.

Wounds in Intestines

Those who do not fully munch their food and have hard things in the meals, that too at irregular hours, suffer from this problem. To heal up the wounds in intestines, quince or quince seeds are ideal to heal up these wounds. Just eat a spoonful of these grains and allow them to get dissolved in your mouth. The saliva would be quite thick like gum. You must continue to suck these grain and in a couple of days these wounds of intestines would heal up. But during this period take no solid food.

Weak Eye-sight

Extract the juice of two small and juicy, sweet oranges, add a little of black pepper powder and drink the juice in the afternoon, preferably about two hours after your lunch. But one or two doses would not give the desired relief. Continue the treatment for about one and a half months to get back your powerful eye-sight.

Acidity

The easiest and tried and tested remedy to cure acidity to have as much cucumber or kakadis as one can without sprinkling salt over it. For if you sprinkle salt over them, you again use something which adds to the acidity. After you have eaten your normal meal, don't drink water over it but have kakadis or cucumber. You can also have them with your food.

19

General Properties of Fruits & Vegetables

Fruits are one of the oldest forms of food known to man. Fresh and dry fruits are the natural staple food of man. They contain substantial quantities of essential nutrients in a rational proportion. They are excellent sources of minerals, vitamins and enzymes. They are easily digested and exercise a cleaning effect on the blood and the digestive tract. Persons on this natural diet will always enjoy good health. Fresh and dry fruits are thus not only a good food but also a good medicine.

FRUITS

Fruits have highly benefecial effect on this human system. The main physiological actions of fruits are as follows:

Hydrating Effect

Taking of fruits or fruit juice is the most pleasant way of hydrating the organism.The water absorbed by sick persons in this manner has an added advantage of supplying sugar and minerals at the same time.

Diuretic Effect

Clinical observations have shown that postassium, magnesium and sodium contents of the fruit act as a diuretic and diuresis frequency of urination is considerably increased when fruits and fruit juice are taken. They lower the urine density and thereby accelerate the elimination of nitrogenous waste and chlorides.

Alkalinising Effect

The organic acids of the salts in fruits produce alkaline carbonates, when transformed within the organism, which alkalise the fluids. All fruits promote intestinal elimination. This keeps the body free from toxic wastes which creep into the blood from an overloading, sluggish intestinal tract.

Mineralisig Effect

Fruits furnish minerals to the body. Dried fruits such as apricots, raisins and dates are rich in calcium and iron. These minerals are essential for strong bones and good blood respectively.

Laxative Effect

The fibrous matter in fruits, cellulose aids in the smooth passage of the food in the digestive tract and easy bowel action. Regular use of fruits prevents and cures constipation.

Tonic Action

Fruits, as dependable sources of vitamins, exert a tonic effect in the body. Guavas, custard apples and citrus fruits, like lemons and oranges are particularly valuble sources of vitamin C. These fruits are usually eaten fresh and raw, thus making the vitamins fully available to us. Several fruits contain good amounts of carotene which gets converted to vitamin A in the body. A medium-sized mango can provide as much as 15,000 international units of vitamin A which is sufficient for full one week and this vitamin can be stored in the body. The common papaya is an excellent source of vitamin C and carotene.

Fruits are at their best when eaten in the raw and ripe state. In cooking, they lose portions of the nutrient salt and corbohydrates. They are most beneficial when taken as a separate meal by themselves, preferably for breakfast in the morning.

Medicinal Properties of Fruits

Moreover certain fruits can combat specific aliments. It should, however, be remembered that in the therapeutic use of any fruit as a treatment for specific disease, nothing except that particular fruit or its juice should be taken in the system at the time of treatment. Thus when utilising lemon juice as a food remedy, the juice should be taken in the system at the time of treatment. Thus when utilising lemon juice as a food remedy, the juice should be taken at least half an hour before consuming any other food.

It has been found that fruit sugars, calcium, iron, vitamins A, B complex and C control the gradation of heart energy. Hence, eating fruit like apple, lemon, orange and pomegranate can aid the proper functioning of the heart and keep it healthy even in old age.Fruits like apple,date and mango have direct action on the central nervous system. The phosphorus, glutamic acid and vitamins A and B complex of these fruits exert a protective and tonic effect on the nervous exhaustion, mental tension, hysteria and insomnia.

All berries being extremely rich in iron, phosphorus and sodium, are highly beneficial for blood building and nerve strengthening. Lemon can be good food remedy in case of liver ailments, indigestion and rheumatism. Watermelons are the best kidney cleansers. The water flushes through the kidneys and traces of various minerals contained in the water act as healilng agents.

The soothing qualities of pineapple and pomegranates are helpful in catarrh, hay fever and other chronic nasal and bronchial aliments. The common cold may be treated with grapefruit juice. This juice helps cure the infection by activating the orange of elimination.

Fresh and fully ripe fruits like grapes, apples, bananas and figs are best suited for all brain defeciencies. They contain a superior quality of easily digestible sugar which is transformed into physical energy that refreshes the brain. Walnut is a positive remedy for weakness of the brain.

CLASSIFICATION OF FRUITS

Simple Fleshy Fruits

One of the major types of simple fleshy fruits is the berry. The term 'berry' is applied to pulpy fruits like tomatoes, grapes, blueberries. Leathery skinned fleshy fruits are orange, limes, grape fruits etc. Hard skinned fleshy fruits are cucumbers and melons.

The second major type of fleshy fruit is the drupe or stone fruit like cherry, peach and olive.

Simple Dry Fruits

Simple dry fruits are dehiscent or indehiscent. Dehiscent fruits open when matured to release the seeds. Indehiscent fruits remain closed throughout the period of their development. Dehiscent fruits are pea and bean. Indehiscent fruits are butter-cup and buck wheat.

Compound Fruits

There are two general types of compound fruits, viz, aggregate and multiple fruits, each of which is the product of two or more pistils in one flower. They are strawberries, raspberries and blackberries.

Multiple Fruits

They sometimes look superficially like aggregate fruits but these are products of many separate flowers that unite into a fleshy, closely packed mass as they mature. The mulberry, pineapple, breadfruit and the orange are good example of multiple fruits.

VEGETABLES

Vegetables are natural sources of essential and valuable nutrients. They help the body to endurance, in repairing its defective metabolism, in repairing tissues and, in building up energy. They are rich in vitamins, minerals, roughage and cleansing process. Nature has its lap, variety of vegetables, which are important and essential factors to various needs of human body. Even animals live and thrive on vegetables and herb's to feed and cure themselves. For every living being nature has plenty of variety to offer. They are available in the form of seed, roots, stems, leaves and fruits. Group of vitamin B-complex, iron, protein, carbohydrates can be found in plenty from various vegetables. But calcium and vitamin E are quite low in them.

How to Use Vegetable

All leafy and green vegetables are essential part of our diet and to derive optimum benefits, they should be used in their raw fresh form, as is done in case of preparing salads. For preparing a nutritious and tasty salad, it is essential that they should be green, fresh, leafy, dry and crisp, so as to satiate our taste buds and also to build up body's resistance, in addition to supplying essential nutrients. In case vegetables are required to be cooked (which should be avoided, as far as possible) following points, if kept in mind, will go along way in the preservation of their nutrients values.

1. Vegetables should always be used fresh and washed thoroughly. After washing them properly in water, they should be cut into large pieces, they should not be washed again, as it would take away all their nutrient values.
2. Avoid frying or cooking vegetables as cooking and heating destroy their food values.
3. It is advisable to boil, instead of deep-frying or cooking the cut vegetables and, for boiling purposes a cooker should be used so that the vegetables do not lose advantage of stem. Put some water (sufficient enough to immerse and soak the vegetables) in the cooker and some salt to it. When the salted water reaches its boiling point, insert the cut vegetables into it so that vegetables do not stay in the steam and hot water for longer period. This way, B Complex and vitamin ' C ' can be preserved to the maximum.
4. Use only that quantity of water, which will suffice to cover the vegetables, because the more the water the more the time consumed for softening or for reducing them into pulp. Certain vegetables like spinach, leafy vegetables and tomatoes, have enough of natural water, hence there is no need to add any extra amount of water to them for cooking.
5. Climatic change and exposures should not affect quality of vegetables. Keeping the vegetables in the refrigerators is not recommended. Purchase the vegetable which could suffice for one or two meal servings. Always purchase fresh vegetables.
6. Vegetables should be boiled to the extent that their natural colour and flavor remains intact.
7. Vegetables after been cooked, should always be served

fresh and hot. Fringe and cooked vegetables do lose most of their food value and taste.

8. As far as possible, vegetables should be steam boiled in their natural juices (water) on very slow fire and after cooking, do not throw (away) or drain away their water, thus allowing the vegetables to use their own natural water or juice.
9. Unless the skin of a vegetable is too hard to be chewed, it should not be separated/peeled off.
10. For steaming/boiling purpose, never use any aluminum utensil, as aluminum is a soft metal and is amenable to bad effect of alkalies and food acid, as such powerful astringent properties of aluminum harm immensely soft lining of the stomach, causing various digestive disorders.

Normally a person taking around 300 gms of vegetables per day would stay in sound health. Out of this 120 gms should be in the form of leafy vegetables, about 90—100 gms in the form of ladyfingers, brinjals etc., and the rest of 90 gms in the form of tubers and roots.

NUTRITIONAL, THERAPEUTIC AND MEDICINAL USES

Vitamins in Vegetables

(i) Vitamin 'A' is essential for health of skin, better eyesight, for avoiding or delaying night blindness and for providing a protective shield against infarctions to minimize the risk of catching cold. It is, thus, prophylactic for various digestive skin, eye, and respiratory tract infections. Vitamin 'A' is found in plenty in papaya, carrots, leafy vegetables, yellow pumpkin and tomatoes (rich sources of carotene). In short, orange coloured and deep green, yellow coloured vegetables are rich sources of carotene.

(ii) Fresh and green turnips, fenugreek leaves and beet contains maximum amount of riboflavin, the deficiency of which can cause stomatitis, cracking of lip corners, eczema, premature wrinkled face. Riboflavin is also necessary for general health and growth of hair, eyes, skin and nails.

It is always preferable and better to obtain these vitamins B—2 (of B—complex vitamin group) from all available natural resources, rather than depending on inorganic substances.

Vitamin—C (Asborsic acid) is required for growth, repair and upkeep tissues and joints, their normal functioning not excluded, for healthy teeth and gum to build up and sustain normal resistance of the body to various impending infections. Deficiency of ascorbic acid may cause anemia, premature aging, and scurvy, bleeding the gums, promote to multiple infections. It is available in good quantity from cabbage, drumstick leaves, spinach, Indian gooseberry, bitter ground, lemon, tomato as far as possible should always be had from fresh vegetables, instead of rotten, stale and withered vegetables. Those, who smoke regularly, say 5-10 or even more cigarettes a day, are advised to use at least juice of lemon in any form they prefer in the absence thereof, a daily dose of 200-250 mg of Vitamin—C.

Minerals

Iron, copper, potassium, magnesium, manganese and calcium are essential minerals which help to maintain electrolytic balances in the body and also help fats, proteins carbohydrates, generated by food to get absorbed the body. Excess of salt and liquids are also eliminated through excretory organs of the body. To seek relief or atleast, in amelioration of symptons in cases of Nephritis (swelling of kidneys) edema, swelling in heart and renal affections, diuretic action is very important and this action is promoted and prompted by beans, radish, turnip, brinjal, potatoes and spinach. For patients of kidney stones, spinach is a forbidden vegetable as also use of tomatoes in any form.

All minerals are essential nutrient factors and are present in our body in very negligible proportions but even then, their presence, utility and efficiency can not be denied. Fortunately, our food meets all the requirements of the above mentioned minerals, but iron and calcium are the two most important minerals, as iron is required for formation of blood in anemia of the emaciated, malnourished underfed. Hemoglobin is an indispensable constituent of blood, which helps in carrying oxygen to cells in various parts of the body. Rich sources of calcium and iron are carrot, tomato, fenugreek leaves, bitter ground, spinach and beetroot.

Juice of Vegetables

Like fruit juices, vegetable juices are equally important for the body. Vegetable juices can provide elements and enzymes for all tissues and cells of the body. If one opts to choose fresh juices of vegetables, in place of raw ones, one can be rest assured that one's assimilative and digestive process can be bettered and improved upon. Juices obtained from leafy green vegetables, such as spinach, tomatoes, cucumber, lettuce, celery and cabbage are no less nutritious than fruit juices, apart from juices extracted from carrot, raddish, beetroot, onion and potato. In order to get optimum mileage, certain fruits and vegetables can be mixed but, preference should always be given to mixing of juices of vegetables with green leafy vegetables, juices of root vegetables and leafy (green) vegetables should be better combined and mixed.

Vegetable juices ignite and promote appetite for this purpose, its intake should always be proceed before diet but when the need to digest the ingested diet is felt, it should always be followed after diet. This way vegetable juices serve twin purpose. Certain juices of vegetables are exclusively needed at times, for curing certain ailments.

For removal of constipation, green leafy vegetables (like salad, sarson ka saag and palak) juices of cabbage, carrot, turnip, beet, radish, mint, lemon, ginger and garlic, aided by slight amount of salt (preferably black salt), will go a long way in curing of even habitual and obstinate constipation. Triphala is another useful combination of herbs. It should be taken daily with lukewarm water or hot water or hot milk, at the time of retiring to bed. It must be ensured that plenty of roughage and bulking agent are taken to render intestines mobile. Even habitual and regular use in the morning on empty stomach, of lemon juice mixed with lukewarm water, will remove chronic constipation.

20

Home Treatment by Water

Water is panacea for chronic and incurable diseases. Rise early from bed. Do not wash your face and mouth as you do normally. Sit comfortably and drink four large glasses of water. Do not take any thing for 45 minutes. You can wash your face and brush your mouth after drinking water.

Always drink water after an hour of breakfast and meals. Regular intake of water in early morning gives relief in following diseases:

1. Diabetes
2. Acne, Boils
3. Headache
4. Blood pressure
5. Old age and wrinkles
6. Arthritis
7. Paralysis problem of ladies
8. Anaemia
9. Heart diseases, Faintness
10. Cold, Cough, Asthma, Bronchitis
11. Obesity
12. Meningitis
13. Disorders of liver
14. Tuberculosis
15. Disorders of the eye
16. Irregular menstruation
17. Urinary problems, Stones, etc.
18. Hyperacidity Asthma, Bronchitis
19. Gastric trouble and diseases concerned with back, Spine
20. Cancer of ovary
21. Swelling, Fever
22. Digestive disorders
23. Piles
24. Diseases caused by Vata, Pitta, Cough.

25. Mental weakness, etc.

If sick persons or soft natured persons with a delicate physique are unable to take four glasses of water at a stretch, they should start from one or two glasses and then gradually they should start taking four glasses. Take four glasses of water regularly. Experiments have proved that different diseases can be cured within the time given below by its regular use:

Hypertension	—	Within one month
Gastric trouble	—	Within ten days
Cancer	—	Within six months
Constipation	—	Within ten days
Diabetes	—	Within one month
Leucorrhoea	—	Within one month

Other diseases described above may be cured within four to six months according to their nature. Drinking four glasses of water does not have any ill-effects on health. Only urge to pass urine will be great and you will pass urine in large quantities frequently. Passing of stool will be easy and complete. It will facilitate the expulsion of the accumulated waste matter very effectively and leave you fresh. Besides hydrotherapy certain other measures or house hold remedies are also advised for such disorders.

Some Important Facts

1. Never drink water before passing urine or just after passing urine.
2. Passing urine after meals prevents formation of stones.
3. Stand on forefoot and then pass urine. This posture prevents formation of stones.
4. Water contained in copper vessel is hundred times more useful.
5. Take juice of one lemon in a glass of warm water before going to bed. It gives relief in coryza.
6. Take juice of one lemon and teaspoon of honey in warm water in morning. It helps in curing obesity and improves complexion.

7. In early morning, chew five leaves of Neem (Azadiracta indica) and tulsi (Ocimum basilium) and drink a glass of water after chewing these leaves. This can prevent you from carcinoma (Cancer) and plague too.
8. Take a little rice (raw-one or two tea spoons) with a glass of water to cure liver disorders.
9. The water kept in a shankh for a whole night is remedy for stammering speech. Continue this for four to six months.

Role of Water on Stomach

There is secretion of stomachic juice in stomach to digest food. The more genuine the stomachic juice, the better digestion of food.

If someone takes liquid whether it is water, wine or beer, the stomachic juice will not remain genuine. It would be adulterated by the intake of water, wine or beer and would not be effective in digestion of food.

Similarly, if some person takes water six or eight times while taking his meal, it would liquidate stomachic juice so much that it would not be able to act as digestive juice.

Do not take water at all during meals. If you have to take it, take very small quantity of it, so that genuine stomachic juice may be absorbed in all eaten food.

If you feel thirsty after one hour or more of taking food, please take water in limited quantity. Body especially stomach needs water at interval from time to time to liquidate its juice, to increase its quantity and to absorb the solid material (food). The body itself informs whenever it needs it. Sometimes, the desire to take water is slow and sometimes it is very fast. One should be particular about intake whether it is from healthy or sick stomach. One should take it as much as it is sufficient and good for health.

It should be taken at equal intervals of time especially when one is suffering from fever. One should not take a glass of water at a stretch but each five or ten minutes in less quantity. Intake of water at a stretch by a patient of fever, will not quench his thirst, rather it would increase other symptoms of illness.

Water taken in less quantity is at once accepted and absorbed by stomach. Repetition of its intake at each half-an-hour produces juice in more quantity and removes whole dullness and constipation by flowing in body and intestines. It cools them also.

One can use luke-warm water or cold water according to its taste.

Use of Water

1. Saline water is necessary in dehydration caused by cholera, fever, diabetes, diarrhoea, etc.
2. It is useful to take water with salt, sugar, lemon and honey. Patients of kidney diseases should use water with salt in supervision of some naturopath.
3. Some vegetables, water of pulse, sharbat of lemon and juice etc. contain water. They give us minerals and salts along with water.

21

Herbal Tips

Here are some herbal recipes which can be tried by anyone.

Haemoglobin

Prepare leafy vegetables in an iron kadai. It will taste good. The kadai is a good source of iron which is required to increase haemoglobin in blood.

Constipation

a. The best way to deal with constipation it to change food habits. Milk boiled vegetables, fruits and their juices should be taken in large quantities, together with foods containing a lot of roughage and fibrous matters.

b. 10 g of senna leaves and 5 g of aniseed should be boiled in a cup of water with sugar, then strained and drunk before retiring for the night.

c. Half a litre of milk mixed with 50 g of khand taken at night will give relief.

d. Another remedy is to eat 40 g of gulkand with milk everyday.

e. If these remedies fail to give relief, 6 g of the rind of harr should be finely powdered and mixed with a little luke warm and salt be taken.

f. Take bathu ka saag during the season for getting rid of obstinate constipation.

Toothache

a. A paste made of finely ground leaves of tulsi should be warmed a little and applied to the aching tooth.

b. Ginger ground into a paste with a pinch of salt also relieves toothache.

c. Applying clove oil is also effective.

d. Brush your teeth with dried, powdered leaves of tulsi to strengthen gums and prevent pain and pyrrohoea.

e. Brush your teeth after each meal to keep away dental problems.

f. Avoid chewing tobacco, pan-masala and other similar items to avoid early decay.

g. Wash and dry neem leaves; grind them to a fine powder. Sprinkle this powder over the toothpaste before brushing your teeth. You will never have complaints of tooth decay or any mouth diseases.

(A) For Vigour

Onion juice	...	2 tsp
Honey	...	2 tsp
Adrak juice	...	1 tsp

To be taken twice, morning and evening for ten or fifteen days.

(B) For Vigour and strength

Onion juice	...	2 tsp
Honey	...	2 tsp
Desi-ghee	...	2 tsp
Egg yolk	...	1 tsp

Mix the above materials and warm it on stove, add mishri and take once in the morning for 15 days.

Leucoderma or White Spot on Skin

(if it is senseless, it could be leprosy then do not use this prescription).

Eat bathu ka sag daily during the season in form of roti or dal-sag and use its juice over spots daily at least 2/3times. Eat anjir regularly for a month.

For Malaria

Tulsi	...	10 leaves
Bhang	...	5 leaves
Kali-mirch	...	10-15 pieces

Grind the above mixture to a paste and make pea size pellets. Dry it in shake. Two pellets three times a day.

For Nausea

(a) Neebu-pani at the time of nausea will be helpful.

(b) Soft kheera should be eaten gradually to get rid of obstinate nauseatic condition.

For Purifying Blood

A plant commonly called Mundi, its aqueous extract (one cup) daily purifies the blood.

For Angina and Ischaemic Heart Disease

1. Puskarmula
2. Arjun
3. Kut
4. Proshnaparini
5. Guggulu

Above plants are equally powdered and 10g powder is left ovenight in a cup of water and taken in the morning.

Fever/Headache/Bodyache/Malaria

1.	Ghiraita	...	5 leaves
2.	Neem leaves	...	5 leaves
3.	Tulsi	...	10 leaves
4.	Lemon Grass	...	5 leaves
5.	Black pepper	...	10-15 pieces

Mix all, boil and strain, add sugar to taste. Take half cup 3 times a day.

DYSENTERY/TENUSMUS/DIARRHOEA

(a) Grind whole plant of duddhi in water. Strained water extract (half cup) if taken 2/3 times a day gives quick relief.

For cold

Tulsi ... 10 leaves

Honey ... 2 tsp

Make paste of leaves and mix with honey. Taken in the morning, it will keep out cold and cough away and will also help in bringing down blood pressure.

Eczema

(a) Apply garlic juice and lemon juice to the affected place. It will clear fungus infection.

(b) Eczema/fungus infection of nails, hand and feet will be cleared with the use of Mehndi (use continuously for a week). Avoid excess indulgence in water.

(c) Use of tulsi leaves and lemon juice to the infected part will also cure eczema.

High Blood Pressure

(a) 1. Garlic ... 5 cloves

2. Tulsi ... 5 leaves

3. Honey ... 4 tsp

Make a paste of above ingredients and eat it once in the morning without taking anything.

(b) Eat two bananas daily to balance excess sodium in the body. Banana contains enough potassium to cut all effects of sodium (we use as common salt).

Stomach Upsets

1. Tulsi ... 5 leaves
2. Adrak ... Few pieces
3. Black Pepper ... 10-15 pieces

Boil these material. Strain and drink 2/3 times (half cup).

Cough

(a) Dip pieces of one medium sized onion in 10 ml of pure honey, leave it overnight. Remove the pieces and take one spoon juice 3 times a day.

- — Muli as vegetable
- — Anar and angoor juice
- — Liv-52 Tablet, 2 tablet 3 times a day
- — Take rest.

Cuts/Wounds

(a) Sprinkle powdered mehndi or

(b) Sprinkle powdered Haldi.

Arthritis/Gout

(a) Boil mustard oil (10 ml) with one moderate pack of Garlic bulb, apply on the affected parts 3/4 times a day.

(b) Massage with camphor oil 3/4 times a day on the affected parts.

(c) Apply warm mustard oil on the affected parts at the time of bed rest and cover them with dhatura left overnight. Keep doing it for 15 days. Repeat again as per need.

(d) Massage with Turpentine oil/Eucalyptus oil 3/4 times a day on the affected part. Cover that portion with a wet towel and gradually pour hot water (not very hot) from kettle on it.

For Body Resistance to Disease

A mixture of amla, harr, bahera and herb giloya (1:1:1:1) if taken regularly makes the person immune to illness.

To Stop Oozing Blood

Sprinkle Haldi powder, flowing of blood will be stopped.

Hoarse Voice

Sprinkle common salt on the small pieces of adrak. Take the pieces gradually one by one.

Eyebrow

Put a little warm castor oil on scanty eyebrows. This will enhance their growth.

Hair

(a) Extract the juice of the aloe-vera plant and rub it into your scalp. This ensures the healthy growth of hair.

(b) For glowing hair, grind a few whole green grams, lemon peels, a handful of curry leaves and a few "rithas" to a paste and apply to the hair before washing off.

Insect Bite

To cure an insect bit apply any balm on it. It will relieve you of the itchy sensation.

Kidneys

Dry tulsi seeds and grind them with an equal quantity of sugar. One spoon of this powder, taken every morning, is good for the kidney.

Sore Throat

Drink tea with a pinch of pepper to get relief from bad throat.

Skin

Banana is a natural skin whitener. Mash a ripe banana and apply it on the face and neck, and your tan colour will fade away.

Hiccups

Roast some peppercorns and breathe deeply. Your hiccups will stop at once.

Dysentery

A teaspoon of fenugreek seeds in a glass of lukewarm water will bring relief immediately.

Liver

To maintain your liver in a good condition, eat a refrigerated pineapple slice dipped in honey, twice a day.

Hair

A mixture of almond oil, olive oil and castor oil in equal proportions acts as an excellent hair tonic.

Insects

(a) Place neem leaves in your books to prevent them from being attacked by insects.

(b) Burn neem leaves in the courtyard or garden to keep mosquitoes away.

Cold

Drink plenty of lime juice everday as the ascorbic acid (vitamin C) content of lime helps heal wounds quickly, maintain your teeth, helps also hair, nails and complexion in good condition and guard against catching colds.

Nose

Stop nose-bleeds by putting a few drops of pomegranate juice into your nostrils.

Lips

Massage your lips with coriander leaf juice for soft and rosy results.

Eyes

(a) Place cotton wool swabs dipped in cold milk on closed eyes to soothe the eye and remove dark circles.

(b) Triphalla (Amla+Harr+bahera) soaked in water overnight then boiled and filtered. The filtrate to be applied to the eyes along with rose water.

Cough

If you are suffering from a nagging cough or chest congestion, boil three cups water with two fresh betal leaves and four crushed peppercorns, till the water is reduced to half. Strain and drink it every morning and night with a teaspoon of honey added to it.

Medicinal Value of Basil Leaves

(a) For immediate relief from toothache, take two basil leaves, a grain of salt and a pinch of pepper powder and press against the affected tooth.

(b) Mix equal quantities of basil juice, honey, and caraway seed (Ajwain) juice and drink on an empty stomach if you are suffering from cough.

Tea

Tea is a wonderful drink. Brew your tea slowly, it takes three-four minutes for the anti-oxidants to make their way into the water. Anti-oxidants delay ageing.

Motion Sickness

Chewing a couple of cloves while travelling will relieve motion sickness.

High Blood Pressure

If you are suffering from high blood pressure, try this remedy. Boil two cups water with 10 to 15 basil leaves, a few peppercorns and a little sugar. Strain and drink it thrice a day.

Toothache

Take one teaspoon ginger juice, a little edible camphor, a little honey and a pinch of salt. Heat the mixture for a second and apply it on the aching tooth. You will get immediate relief.

Sore Throat

Powder peppercorns and basil leaves and dry them in the shade. Use this powder to make black tea.

Hair Loss

Don't throw away lemon rinds, orange peels and pomegranate skin. Just dry them in the sun and grind to a fine powder. Mix this powder in coconut oil and apply to your hair to prevent hair loss and for glossy hair.

Acidity and Indigestion

Dry roast one teaspoon each of cumin seeds and caraway seeds (ajwain) in a pan. Add one cup water and boil till it is reduced to half its quantity. Strain and add sugar to taste. Drink one teaspoon for relief from acidity and indigestion.

Nausea & Stomach Ailments

Eat a slice of fresh ginger after each meal to protech yourself, from stomach ailments. For immediate relief from nausea, chew salted dry ginger sticks.

Stomach Upsets

For quick relief from an upset stomach, chew a spoonful of 'ajwain' with little black salt.

Cough, Nausea and Vomiting

Take half a cup of onion juice mixed with two teaspoons of honey for relief from cough, nausea and vomiting.

Toxicity

To check if mushrooms are poisonous, boil them in water along with a few garlic flakes. If water turns black they are poisonous.

Enuresis (Passing Urine at Night)

Chewing one teaspoonful of black sesame seeds (til) before going to bed is a sure shot treatment for such problem.

Malnutrition

Banana is a complete food. It has all the ingredients necessary for body's nutrition, growth and strength. So, it is specially recommended for children and old people. But it causes a little bit constipation so, it should be taken with black pepper and salt.

Habitual Abortion

Grind fresh flowers of anar (2g) to a fine paste. Add a little water and filter. Add sugar to taste in filtrate and use it morning and evening (taking 2g flower each time) for three days.

Nausea/Bile

Sharbat of imli cools liver/bile and checks nausea and vomiting especially in summer days. 5 g ripe fruit of imli dipped in water for 1/2 hours, after that it is masticated in water and seeds are thrown out. Now, remaining water containing imli is taken in the afternoon with sugar.

Dropsy/Liver Inflammation

Leaves of kasondi (1g) and Kali mirch (7) is ground together in water and filtered. Filtrate is to be taken morning and evening for one week (each time 1g kasondi and 7 kali mirch).

For all kinds of Fever

Gilo (Gurach)-one gram is powdered and dipped in water. Water is strained and divided in two doses. M'ix each dose with a spoon of sugar and take morning and evening. Better if Ajwain (250mg.) is also added to Gilo.

Face Cream

Chana ka atta (besan)	...	1/2 Cup
Haldi Powder	...	1 tsp
Mustard Oil	...	1/4 to 1/2 Cup

Mix all these materials to a semi-solid paste and apply it on your face. It will bring marvellous glow on your skin. It can be used on hands and legs also.

Cataract

Tobacco leaves	...	1 grams
Arandi ka Tel	...	4 grams

Mix these material to very fine paste and keep it in a small bottle. Apply it to eyes with a rod daily.

Cough

White Pepper	...	1 gram
Misri	...	250 mg

Grind these items to a very fine powder. Now mix it with one tsp malai and take it bit by bit rather lick it gradually.

Fever

Mix equal number of leaves of tulsi, neem and lemon grass plus 7-10 black pepper. Boil it like making tea. Strain the water and drink 3/4 times a day.

Gas/Giddiness

Dhania powder	...	1 gram
Khand	...	250 mg

Mix these two materials in the said ration and keep it in a container, use tsp after each meal with water.

Piles

While going to toilet, put a medium piece of Alum (Fitkari) in water. Use this water after the toilet. Repeat till relief.

Diarrhoea/Indigestion/Gas

Saunf and dhania is to be mixed in equal proportion, powdered and a small amount of misri or khand is added. 2 tsp is to be taken morning and evening. This will stop diarrhoea/indigestion/gas formation and is helpful to eyes.

Eye sight

One small piece of haldi is kept in lemon and when it dries, haldi is taken out and put in fresh lemon and when it dries it is further kept in third/fourth lemon. Now, haldi is ground with one/two drops of water and applied on the eyes with the help of a rod for 7/10 days or as needed.

Cholera

Mix powdered red pepper with honey and prepare fine small pellets (equal to 1/2 pea size). Use 2 pellets when patient feels extreme weakness. It will bring dramatic relief in 2/3 days.

Dog-bite

In case of dog-bite, first apply mustard oil on that part and then pack it with red pepper powder. It will check disease from spreading even if the dog is rabid.

Leprosy

Red Pepper (powdered)	...	1 g
Ghee	...	2.5 g

Mix and keep it in a small container. Use it on the affected part 2/3 times a day. It will bring good results.

Abortion

Tender leaves of babool	...	2 g
Water	...	2 Cups

Boil strain, add mishri to taste. Use this 2/3 days once a day to check abortion.

Dandruff

Add a few drops of ecualyptus oil to the henna mixture before applying it on your hair if you want, dark copper colour. This also helps to get rid of dandruff and leaves your hair shining.

Toothache

For instant relief from severe toothache, press a little turmeric powder into the tooth.

High Blood Pressure

To control high blood pressure, mix equal quantities of onion juice and honey and take one teaspoon every day in the morning.

Diarrhoea

(a) A strong cup of unsweetened black tea is effective in stopping diarrhoea.

(b) Another quick remedy is to peel apple and shred it. Keep the stredded pieces in a plate for approx. 20 minutes until they turn brown in colour, and then eat them.

Constipation

Simply eat a few liquorice sticks. One of its many properties is that it is a natural laxative.

Catarrh

To rid yourself of congestion, mix a teaspoon of vinegar in a glass of warm water and sip frequently.

Coughs

First cut an onion or several flakes of garlic into thin slices. Cover the slices with honey and leaves for two to three hours. Drink a spoonful of the resulting juice throughout the day.

Smelly Feet

Soak your feet in strong tea for 20 minutes every day until smell disappears. To prepare your footbath, brew two tea bags in 500 ml of water for 15 minutes and pour the tea into a basin containing two litres of cool water.

Bleeding Gums

Take lemon juice in a glass of water daily for 3/4 days. Also gargle with salt.

Sprinkle powdered haldi and henna over the oozing blood. This will stop flow of blood immediately.

Chills

Instead of your regular hot tea or coffee, have a glass of hot water mixed with honey and lemon.Put a teaspoon of honey, lemon juice and a little grated ginger in a glass and add hot water stir and drink.

Cracked skin

Apply a mixture of grated potato soaked in olive oil. Leave this for 10 minutes and then rinse off.

Tired Eyes

Lavender oil offers gentle relief for tired for and strained eyes. Add a drop of lavender oil to 500 ml of water and shake the solution well. Dip two cotton wool pads in the liquid, squeeze out the excess water and place one pad over each eyes (Don't use contact lenses at this time).

For General Debility

Sage is an excellent pick-me-up. Take 100g of fresh sage leaves and soak them in a bottle of white wine for two weeks. Add honey for sweetening and leave for an extra 24 hours. Use a muslin cloth for straining, making sure you press as you strain. Collect the solution in a bottle and drink a little before meals.

Spots

Herbs like tea tree oil and lavender oil, both antiseptics, can be applied neatly and quickly to pimples.

Warts

Place some chopped onions in a dish, cover with salt and leave overnight. Twice a day apply the resulting juice to the warts until they disappear.

Bad Breath

Parsley leaves are rich in chlorophyll, nature own deodoriser. Chew some leaves regularly and your breath will remain fresh. Alternatively, you can chew some cardamom seeds to sweeten your breath.

Indigestion

Place a teaspoon of freshly grated ginger into a pan and add a cup of water. Cover and allow to simmer for 5 minutes. Strain the contents and drink.

Nausea

Powered cinnamom and sliced ginger work by interrupting nausea signals sent from the stomach to the brain. If you are a herbal tea drinker, simply sprinkle powdered cinnamom on the tea and drink ginger-tea to check nausea.

Nose Bleeds

Dip a cotton bud in rose water and dab it on to the inside of your nostrils to stop the bleeding.

Bruises

Slice a raw onion and place over the bruise. But do not apply this over grave injuries.

Toothache

Cloves are excellent painkillers. You can either chew one, or place it near the tooth. As the juices flow and mix with saliva, they numb the gum and alleviate pain.

Stomach Belches

Eat a small piece of jaggery after eating radish, you can avoid unpleasant belches.

Malaria

Eating a leaf or two of tulsi takes care of many disorders and works wonders during malaria.

Sprain

Add a tsp of salt to two tsp turmeric powder and boil with a little water to obtain a thick paste. Apply while still hot over sprain.

Thirst

Eat a cardamom or two, especially during long journeys, to avoid feeling thirsty.

To Check Bleeding

Sprinkle powdered haldi and henna over the oozing blood. This will stop flow of blood immediately.

Nails

For glossy and strong nails, soak them in a mixture of lemon juice and glycerine.